Healthy Habits FOR

Managing & Reversing Prediabetes

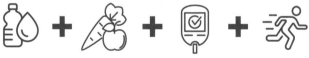

100 Simple, Effective Ways to Prevent and Undo Prediabetes

MARIE FELDMA

Adams Media
New York London Toronto Sydney New Delhi

⚠ adamsmedia

Adams Media
An Imprint of Simon & Schuster, Inc.
57 Littlefield Street
Avon, Massachusetts 02322

First Adams Media trade paperback edition
January 2019

ADAMS MEDIA and colophon are
trademarks of Simon & Schuster.

For information about special discounts for
bulk purchases, please contact Simon &
Schuster Special Sales at 1-866-506-1949 or
business@simonandschuster.com.

The Simon & Schuster Speakers Bureau can
bring authors to your live event. For more
information or to book an event contact
the Simon & Schuster Speakers Bureau at
1-866-248-3049 or visit our website at
www.simonspeakers.com.

Interior design by Heather McKiel

Manufactured in the United States of America

2   2020

Library of Congress Cataloging-in-Publication
Data has been applied for.

ISBN 978-1-5072-0994-3
ISBN 978-1-5072-0995-0 (ebook)

Contains material adapted from the following
titles published by Adams Media, an Imprint
of Simon & Schuster, Inc.: *The Everything®
Guide to Managing and Reversing Pre-Diabetes,
2nd Edition* by Gretchen Scalpi, RD, CDN,
CDE, and Robert Vigersky, MD, copyright
© 2013, ISBN 978-1-4405-5761-3; *The
Everything® Guide to Managing Type 2 Diabetes*
by Paula Ford-Martin with Jason Baker, MD,
copyright © 2013, ISBN 978-1-4405-5196-3;
and *The Everything® Diabetes Book* by Paula
Ford-Martin with Ian Blumer, MD, copyright
© 2004, ISBN 978-1-58062-981-2.

ACKNOWLEDGMENTS

A sincere thanks to Adams Media for providing me with the opportunity to work on this project, which centers on such an important topic. Professionally, I am very grateful to work under David Weingard, who is an inspirational leader to me and all the wonderful staff and clients we work with at Fit4D, where we pride ourselves on making a difference in the lives of those with prediabetes and diabetes. Also, thank you to Dr. David Kayne, a wonderful mentor who has taught me so much about successfully diagnosing and treating prediabetes and diabetes through the patient care and clinical research we have conducted together over the years. In addition, it is with sincere gratitude that I mention my good friend and colleague, fellow dietitian and seasoned chef/author, Cheryl Forberg, who has been very helpful and informative during this entire project.

Many thanks to my husband, Ken—you are my best friend, and I treasure our relationship, in which we motivate and elevate each other every day. I also want to express my heartfelt gratitude to my parents, who have given me ultimate unconditional love and support throughout my life in countless ways. I lovingly acknowledge my daughter, Gabrielle, who inspires me every day to work hard to create a balanced, active, healthy, and happy life for our family. I also appreciate my extended family and friends, along with the readers and supporters of my blog, NourishYouDelicious.Blogspot.com, since its creation nine years ago.

Last but not least, I thank you, the reader, for buying this book and taking the opportunity to take a huge first step in preventing/managing your prediabetes and improving your overall health. I sincerely hope you find this book very useful.

CONTENTS

Part I: Take Control of Your Health and Habits / 9

Part II: Develop Habits for Health / 81

INTRODUCTION

If you are reading this book, odds are that you or someone you know has concerns about prediabetes. And there's cause for concern because one in three adults in the US—approximately *eighty-four million* people—have prediabetes. What's particularly concerning is that up to 90 percent of them don't even know they have it!

The best thing you can do—whether you are worried about developing this condition or have already been diagnosed with it—is develop a set of healthy habits. In this book you'll find one hundred habits that will help you manage—and even reverse—your prediabetes. Even if you don't have the illness and just want to keep up a healthy lifestyle you're already maintaining, these habits can help.

The habits in this book are easy to integrate into your daily routine. For instance:

- Change to eating non-starchy veggies
- Take a daily walk
- Harness the power of deep breathing

See? It's easy! By adopting these simple habits, you can help beat prediabetes.

With these habits in place, you're on your way not only to managing and possibly reversing this disease; you've also adopted a healthier lifestyle that will make you feel better in every way. You'll understand the importance of your lifestyle choices and how to make those changes last.

If you're already doing things that are good for your health, you'll see how to maintain them and turn them into routines.

Now let's get started with healthy habits for managing and rolling back prediabetes.

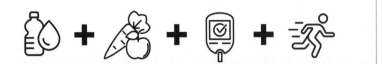

PART I
Take Control of Your Health and Habits

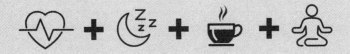

Chapter 1

Prediabetes: What It Is and How to Treat It

LET'S START BY learning and understanding more about prediabetes, how it affects your body, and how it differs from diabetes, as well as how it is diagnosed. Once you know that, you can work with your medical team and others to get started on a set of healthy habits to treat it.

The Pancreas: A Key Player in the Endocrine System

The endocrine system is composed of glands that secrete the hormones. These travel through the circulatory system to regulate metabolism, growth, sexual development, and reproduction. The glands that make up the endocrine system include the adrenals, the thyroid and parathyroid, the hypothalamus, the pituitary, the pineal, the reproductive glands (testes, ovaries), and the pancreas. If any of these glands secrete either too little or too much of a hormone, the entire body can be thrown off-balance. Diabetes mellitus is classified as a disease of the endocrine system, so understanding how the pancreas functions as part of this system can help illustrate the way diabetes and prediabetes develop.

The pancreas is located in the abdomen, next to the upper part of the small intestine. It's long and tapered with a thicker bottom end (or head), which is cradled in the downward curve of the duodenum—a part of the small intestine. The long end (or tail) of the pancreas extends up behind the stomach toward the spleen. A main duct, or channel, connects the pancreas to the duodenum.

A Tale of Two Functions

The pancreas performs two major functions in the body, which are carried out by two different types of cells located within the organ. These cells allow it to pull double duty as both a digestive organ and a regulator of energy balance and metabolism. Sitting behind the stomach, the spongy pancreas secretes both digestive enzymes and endocrine hormones. Taking a closer look at the physiology of the pancreas involves distinguishing between its exocrine tissue and the endocrine cells and their actions.

The exocrine tissue of the pancreas is a group of specialized cells that secrete digestive enzymes into a network of ducts that join the main pancreatic duct and end up in the duodenum. There the enzymes are key in processing carbohydrates, proteins, and other nutrients. In essence, the exocrine portion of the pancreas is primarily involved with digestion.

The other group of cells is the pancreatic endocrine tissue. For all intents and purposes, the endocrine part of the pancreas is the one to watch as far as prediabetes and diabetes are concerned. The endocrine pancreas actually accounts for a very small anatomical part of the organ, and it contains key cell clusters known as islets of Langerhans. These islets are constructed of various cell types, and each cell type makes and secretes a different hormone. The three main and most well studied include:

- Alpha cells: These manufacture and release glucagon, a hormone that raises blood glucose levels.
- Beta cells: These monitor blood sugar levels and produce glucose-lowering insulin in response.
- Delta cells: These produce the hormone somatostatin, which researchers believe is responsible for directing the action of both the beta and alpha cells.

Islets of Langerhans: What's in a Name?

These islets (pronounced EYE-lets) are named after Dr. Paul Langerhans, a German physician who first described them in medical literature in 1869. A normal human pancreas can contain as many as one million islets, yet they amount to just about 1–2 percent of the total mass of the pancreas.

The Liver's Important Partnership with the Pancreas

Located toward the front of the abdomen and above the stomach, the liver is the center of glucose storage. This important organ converts glucose—the fuel that the cells of the human body require for energy—into its principal storage form, glycogen. Glycogen is warehoused in muscle and in the liver itself, where it can later be converted back to glucose for energy with the help of the hormones epinephrine (secreted by the adrenal glands) and glucagon (from the alpha cells of the pancreas). Together, the liver and pancreas preserve a delicate balance of blood glucose and insulin, produced in sufficient amounts to both fuel cells and maintain glycogen storage.

Insulin and Blood Sugar

While the liver is one source of glucose, most of the glucose the body uses is manufactured from food, primarily carbohydrates. Cells then convert blood glucose for energy. Insulin is the hormone that makes it all happen. As previously mentioned, insulin is a hormone produced and secreted by the beta cells of the pancreas, which is a key to help regulate blood sugar. When you eat a meal containing carbohydrates, they are broken down to glucose in the blood. Often referred to as "carbs," carbohydrates include starchy foods such as bread, rice, pasta, sweets, and some fruit. The increase in your blood glucose, a.k.a. "blood sugar," signals the pancreas to release insulin, and this hormone allows the sugar to move from the blood into cell tissues, such as the muscles, fat cells, and the liver, where it can be used for energy or stored as glycogen or fat.

To visualize the role of insulin in the body and in diabetes, think of a flattened basketball. The ball needs air (or glucose) to supply the necessary energy to bounce. To fill a basketball, you insert an inflating needle into the ball valve to open it, then pump air into the ball. Likewise, when a cell needs energy, insulin binds to an insulin receptor, or cell gateway, to "open" the cell and let glucose in for processing. You can blow pounds and pounds of compressed air at the ball valve, but without a needle to open it, the air will not enter. The same applies to your cells. Without insulin to bind to the receptors and open the cell for glucose, the glucose cannot enter. Instead, it builds up to damaging levels in the bloodstream.

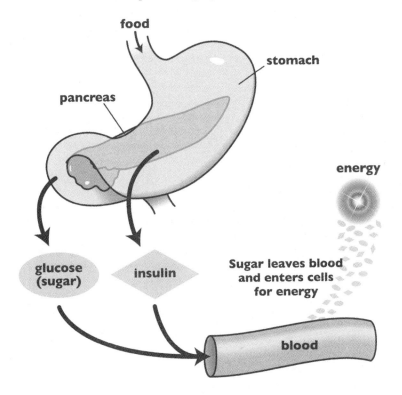

How it works: the pancreas, glucose, and insulin. Normally, insulin enters the bloodstream to regulate the levels of glucose.

What Goes Wrong in Prediabetes and Diabetes?

In people with prediabetes and eventually type 2 diabetes, the inflating needle (the insulin) is the wrong size or shape for the valve (the insulin receptor), or the valve itself is too small or missing. This phenomenon, where there's plenty of insulin but the body isn't using it properly, is known as insulin resistance. As the beta cells try to produce more and more insulin in an effort to compensate for the body's growing inability to process glucose, another problem occurs. The pancreatic beta cells start to "burn out" and die, and insulin insufficiency (also known as insulin deficiency) is the result. The actual mechanics of how this occurs, and how early it happens in type 2, is not completely understood. But researchers have hypothesized that those who have progressed to type 2 diabetes at diagnosis may have lost as much as 90 percent of their beta cell function.

Blood Sugar Control: Why Is It So Important?

Keeping your blood sugars under control is key to managing prediabetes and preventing adverse outcomes, such as the development of type 2 diabetes and all the potential complications that can go with it. A diagnosis of prediabetes does not mean you will automatically develop type 2 diabetes. If you take action early to get the right treatment to return blood sugars to normal range, you can avoid diabetes. However, the longer you let your blood sugars stay elevated, the greater your risk of progressing to type 2 diabetes.

The pancreas of a person who is on the fringe of type 2 diabetes generates insulin, but the body is unable to process it in sufficient amounts to control blood sugar levels. This inability is due to a problem with how the body's cells—specifically the insulin receptors that attract and process the hormone—recognize and use insulin. As blood sugar levels rise, the pancreas pumps out more and more insulin to try to compensate. This pumped insulin may bring blood sugar levels down to a degree, but it also results in high levels of circulating insulin, a condition known as hyperinsulinemia. At a certain threshold, the weakened pancreas cannot produce enough insulin, and over time beta cell mass is lost. As beta cells die, insulin deficiency develops. At this point, you move into type 2 diabetes. If you don't carefully control your blood sugars at this point, then both short- and long-term complications can develop.

Diabetes Control Reduces Complications

Results from a ten-year landmark clinical study, the Diabetes Control and Complications Trial (DCCT), revealed the importance of blood sugar control in helping prevent diabetic complications. The research, conducted by the National Institute of Diabetes and Digestive and Kidney Diseases (NIDDK), which concluded in 1993, showed that type 1 diabetic participants who kept their glucose levels close to normal lowered their chances of developing complications with their eyes, kidneys, and nerves. It led to many follow-up trials that helped develop treatment standards for patients with type 1 and 2 diabetes. These treatments encourage good blood sugar control to improve longevity and quality of life.

Short-Term Problems with Elevated Blood Sugars

The human body needs glucose to function, but too much glucose circulating in the bloodstream has the potential to be toxic to all the tissues and organs of the body, including the insulin-producing beta cells of the pancreas. This is known as glucotoxicity. When insulin isn't available, blood sugar levels rise higher and higher in the bloodstream. If you've got this condition, you may experience fatigue, excessive thirst, and increased urination. In the short term, if blood sugars are not controlled, you can develop the three Ps: polydipsia (increased thirst), polyuria (increased urination), and polyphagia (increased hunger). These are the classic symptoms many people develop before receiving a diabetes diagnosis. Blurred vision and skin changes such as acanthosis nigricans (areas of darkened and thickened skin) can also develop early on.

Alert! Look Out for Acanthosis Nigricans

Acanthosis nigricans is one of the few early signs of prediabetes. It is characterized by a darkening of skin that typically affects the neck, armpits, elbows, knees, or knuckles. The darkening of pigment around these areas of the body can be an early sign of glucose abnormality. The condition doesn't affect everyone and is found most often in Native Americans, African Americans, and Hispanics. While there is no specific treatment for acanthosis nigricans, treatment of underlying conditions, such as a glucose abnormality, may restore some of the normal color to affected areas of skin.

If blood sugar levels continue to rise and become very elevated, serious acute complications can develop. A severe rise in blood sugar can result in diabetic ketoacidosis (DKA) or hyperosmolar hyperglycemic nonketotic coma (HHNC)—both are life-threatening medical emergencies.

Diabetic Ketoacidosis

DKA occurs when the body does not have enough insulin available to use glucose, the body's normal source of energy. When cells don't get the glucose they need, the body will begin to burn fat for energy instead, and this process produces ketones. These are chemicals the body creates when it breaks down fat to use for fuel. When ketones build up in the blood, they make it more acidic. When levels get too high, you can develop DKA. Although DKA can happen to anyone with diabetes, it is rare in those with type 2.

Hyperosmolar Hyperglycemic Nonketotic Coma

A more frequent complication in type 2 diabetics, mainly in the elderly, is hyperosmolar hyperglycemic nonketotic coma (HHNC). HHNC tends to occur in people with very high blood sugars when something else is going on in their bodies. This can include an illness or infection. When blood sugars are very high, the excess blood sugar spills over into the urine, since the body is trying to get rid of it. Initially, people suffering from HHNC tend to go to the bathroom a lot. If they don't consume enough fluids, eventually they become dehydrated. They will make fewer trips to the bathroom, but that's because the body is making little or no urine. Severe dehydration will lead to seizures, coma, and eventually death. HHNC may take days or even weeks to develop.

Long-Term Consequences of Blood Sugars Gone Out of Control

Over longer periods of time, elevated blood sugars can damage virtually all the systems of the body. Chronically high blood sugars can lead to blood vessel and nerve damage, which can result in:

- Cardiovascular disease, namely increased risk of heart attack or stroke
- Nerve damage in areas such as the hands and feet and problems with the nerves that control the bladder, the intestines, and the genitals
- Eye problems such as retinal eye disease, cataracts, and glaucoma
- Kidney problems ranging from early-stage microalbuminuria (protein in the urine) to progressive decrease in kidney function and ultimately end-stage renal disease in which the kidneys no longer function and dialysis or a transplant is needed
- Skin problems such as dry or itchy skin and bacterial or fungal infections
- Foot issues such as calluses, foot ulcers, poor circulation, and amputation (circulatory problems can lead to amputation of not just the feet but also parts of the leg above or below the knee)
- Gastrointestinal disturbances, namely gastroparesis, where the stomach empties too slowly
- Mental health issues such as depression and stress, which are more common in type 2 diabetes
- Sexual function problems, including erectile dysfunction in men and vaginal dryness in women

Why You Shouldn't Ignore Prediabetes

Not that long ago, doctors did not routinely screen for, or treat, prediabetes aggressively. People who had glucose readings that were higher than normal but were not yet diabetic were seldom advised to reduce their risk of developing type 2 diabetes. That was before there was a good understanding about how glucose levels in the prediabetic range could actually cause vascular damage or other complications. Prediabetes is a danger in itself: it increases the likelihood of stroke and heart disease by 50 percent! Today we know that waiting until someone has progressed to diabetes can mean that complications have already begun to take hold. For this reason, doctors have lowered the fasting blood glucose cutoff for prediabetes from 140 mg/dl (milligrams per deciliter) to 125 mg/dl. Today, a normal fasting blood glucose is below 100 mg/dl.

The lowering of the blood glucose range cutoffs has helped detect poor glucose tolerance in many people much earlier. If you've been informed that you have prediabetes, you can be grateful that you know about the problem now, at an early stage. The most compelling reason to address prediabetes is your ability to halt or slow the progression to diabetes. If the right things are done at an early stage, a person may be able to reverse the prediabetic state. Even if you are only able to slow down the eventual progression to diabetes, you can minimize your risk for developing diabetic complications, such as heart disease, kidney failure, or diabetic eye disease.

Keep Blood Sugar Controlled from the Start

People who allow their blood sugar to creep up over time may already be developing some of the complications associated with diabetes. According to the American Diabetes Association, some long-term damage to the body, especially the heart and circulatory system, may already be occurring during prediabetes. Taking actions early on can help you prevent diabetic complications.

Long Term and Short Term

It is important to understand that diabetes does not occur suddenly. For most people, the progression from normal to prediabetic then to diabetic can take a number of years. The longer your body experiences high glucose levels, the greater your chance of developing diabetes-related complications. Keep in mind, timely diagnosis and treatment are important in preventing prediabetes progression and ultimately type 2 diabetes complications in the short and long term.

What Makes Prediabetes Different from Type 2 Diabetes?

The term *prediabetes* was introduced by the American Diabetes Association (ADA) in 2002 as a way to more clearly describe a state that is between normal blood sugar and type 2 diabetes. In the past, your doctor may have diagnosed you with "borderline diabetes." Before 2002, your doctor might have told you (euphemistically), "Your blood sugar is a little high" or "You have a touch of sugar." These words provide little meaning to the person hearing them, and they don't show the urgent need to do something about the situation. Prediabetes is defined by specific boundaries, namely the results of blood glucose tests (described in the next section).

When you have prediabetes, your blood sugar level is higher than normal, but it's not yet high enough to be classified as type 2 diabetes. Prediabetes means that you are on your way to developing diabetes if there are no interventions on your part. *However*—and this is very important to understand—progressing to type 2 diabetes is not inevitable. There is a great deal that you can do to reverse prediabetes and bring your blood sugar level back to a normal range. A diagnosis of type 2 diabetes, on the other hand, is permanent. While there is much that can be done to control diabetes, it is important to realize that type 2 diabetes does not go away.

If you have received a diagnosis of prediabetes, there is some good news. You have received a wake-up call and been given an opportunity to improve your health, lose weight, and make healthy lifestyle changes. If you take action now, you can prevent, or at the very least halt, the progression to a serious, more permanent disease.

Diagnosing Prediabetes

If you are trying to determine whether you have prediabetes or are monitoring your condition after you have been diagnosed, you will need to have some information about your health. This information includes lab tests, blood pressure, and other measurements such as weight and waist circumference. Your prior health history provides additional clues in the determination of prediabetes or diabetes. Three types of blood tests are used to diagnose prediabetes and diabetes:

Fasting Blood Glucose Test

A fasting blood glucose test provides a clue about the possibility of prediabetes. In this simple blood test you draw a sample of blood first thing in the morning after an overnight fast. A fasting blood glucose of 100–125 mg/dl on more than one occasion is an indicator for prediabetes, whereas a fasting blood glucose 126 mg/dl or above indicates diabetes.

Two-Hour Oral Glucose Tolerance Test

Some doctors prefer using a glucose challenge rather than a fasting test. In this case, you are given a glucose drink that provides 75 grams of glucose. Blood is drawn two hours after taking the drink, and then the blood glucose is measured. With this test, a blood glucose result of

140–199 mg/dl two hours after taking 75 grams of glucose (on more than one occasion) indicates prediabetes. Two-hour readings that are above 200 mg/dl on more than one occasion indicate diabetes.

Hemoglobin A1c

When a fasting glucose test or two-hour glucose challenge is done, the reading provides a result for that moment in time. Because your glucose can vary a great deal throughout the day, these tests do not provide information about what your blood sugar is at other times of the day or longer term. That is why a test called the hemoglobin A1c (HbA1c) is done, particularly when your doctor suspects prediabetes or diabetes.

A Fasting Blood Glucose Test Means Just That: *Fasting*

If you are having your blood test in the morning, you should not have anything to eat or drink (besides water) after midnight. Refrain from doing exercise before your test, because that could also affect your reading, providing an inaccurate result.

Hemoglobin is a substance found in red blood cells that carries oxygen from the lungs to all cells in the body. When hemoglobin binds with glucose, an irreversible compound, glycated hemoglobin (or glycohemoglobin), is formed. The A1c portion of glycated hemoglobin is the easiest and largest portion of this compound to measure. A person with higher blood glucose has more glycated hemoglobin than someone with normal blood glucose. Hemoglobin found in red blood cells lasts for sixty to ninety days. As a result, when hemoglobin A1c is measured, the doctor can form a fairly accurate reflection of your average blood glucose levels over the last sixty to ninety days. A hemoglobin A1c between 5.7 percent and 6.4 percent indicates prediabetes and a hemoglobin A1c 6.5 percent and above indicates diabetes.

In addition to checking hemoglobin A1c blood sugar levels and fasting blood glucose levels at diagnosis, your doctor will likely check them at regular intervals thereafter to keep tabs on your progress. Monitoring your hemoglobin A1c and keeping it below 5.7 percent and fasting blood glucose levels close to 100 mg/dl (or more specific targets determined for you individually by your medical team) should be part of your action plan. Your doctor will monitor your hemoglobin A1c and blood sugar levels every three to six months by ordering a blood test and may also want you to check blood sugars at home with the use of a blood glucose meter.

Glucose Meters

If you have been diagnosed with prediabetes, periodically monitoring your own blood sugar with a glucose meter can be a valuable tool to help you track your blood sugar. A glucose meter can be purchased over the counter or prescribed by your doctor. All meters come with easy-to-follow instructions. The readings from the glucose meter will help you learn how different foods affect your blood glucose, or what times of day you may be high or low. You and your doctor can decide how often to check your blood glucose, but two to three times a week may be a good start.

What Other Blood Tests and Measurements Are Important?

Monitoring your blood sugars and HbA1c are just one part of the equation when it comes to keeping your prediabetes in check. There are additional blood tests and other measurements that your medical team may perform to assess your health status. Keeping tabs on your cholesterol, triglycerides, C-reactive protein, and blood pressure are also important.

Cholesterol and Triglycerides

The relationship between cholesterol and heart disease is well known. People with prediabetes or diabetes have more risk for heart disease; therefore, monitoring your cholesterol levels is an important part of your health plan. Knowing your total cholesterol is not sufficient to determine whether you are at risk. You also need to know how much of your total cholesterol represents good cholesterol (HDL, or high-density lipoprotein) or bad cholesterol (LDL, or low-density lipoprotein). Triglycerides, another type of fat found in the blood, are also associated with determining risk factors for heart disease. The following are recommended levels for cholesterol and triglyceride levels for individuals without diabetes or prediabetes. If you have prediabetes, your doctor may want to see readings even lower. This list indicates normal laboratory values for cholesterol and triglycerides.

- Total cholesterol: Less than 200 mg/dl
- LDL cholesterol: Less than 100 mg/dl
- HDL cholesterol: Greater than 40 mg/dl for men; greater than 50 mg/dl for women
- Triglycerides: Less than 150 mg/dl

LDL and HDL levels are much better predictors of heart disease risk than the total cholesterol. Although someone may have a normal total cholesterol reading, they can still be at increased risk if the LDL (bad) cholesterol is higher than recommended levels. If the results of your cholesterol or triglycerides are abnormal, you and your doctor will discuss these results. In addition to lab results, other risk factors such as gender, family history, smoking, weight, and blood pressure help determine the best course of treatment for you. For some individuals, healthy diet, modest weight loss, and a regular exercise plan may be enough to bring cholesterol and triglyceride levels in range. For others, the addition of cholesterol and/or triglyceride-lowering medications may be necessary.

Measure Annually

If your doctor has prescribed cholesterol- or triglyceride-lowering medications for you, a lipid panel, as well as other blood tests, may be required more often to monitor your body's response to the medication. You should have these tests done once a year or more, if required by your doctor.

C-Reactive Protein

C-reactive protein is a protein found in the blood that indicates the amount of inflammation in your body. Inflammation plays a role in prediabetes and diabetes. A high-sensitive C-reactive protein (hsCRP) test can identify low-grade inflammation that increases one's risk for developing heart disease, making this a useful test for people at high risk for heart disease. Elevated CRP levels can also be found in some people with prediabetes or diabetes, or people who are overweight.

Blood Pressure

Just as the prevalence of prediabetes and diabetes is on the rise, having hypertension (high blood pressure) is on the rise as well. Being overweight and having a sedentary lifestyle are two key reasons for an increased prevalence of high blood pressure. Sodium intake in one's diet can be a cause of high blood pressure. The 2010 *Dietary Guidelines for Americans* recommends a reduction in daily sodium intake to less than 2,300 mg. For people who are fifty-one and older, and those of any age who are African American or have hypertension, diabetes, or chronic kidney disease, a further reduction to 1,500 milligrams daily is recommended.

Although the recommendations for sodium intake have been reduced, many people consume much more sodium because they are using convenience, packaged, or processed foods often. Processed food accounts for a large percentage of the sodium Americans consume on a daily basis. If you're salt sensitive, you may develop high blood pressure as a result of high sodium intake. For this reason (as well as others) it's important to read the content labels on packaged food.

Blood pressure is the force of blood against the walls of arteries. The measurement is written one above the other, with the systolic number on top and the diastolic number on the bottom. Systolic blood pressure represents the force with which your heart pumps blood into the arteries. Diastolic blood pressure measures the pressure in the arteries when the heart is at rest, between heartbeats. High blood pressure needs to be treated because continued high pressure exerted on arteries can cause damage to the arteries or the heart. The American College of Endocrinology (ACE) Task Force on the Prevention of Diabetes recommends a target blood pressure of 130/80 for persons with prediabetes. This is the same target for persons with diabetes.

Weight, Body Mass Index, and Waist Circumference

Monitoring your weight is key to managing your prediabetes. Excess weight and obesity (determined by the body mass index) can contribute to your problems with your body's ability to use its own insulin, high blood pressure, and elevated cholesterol/triglycerides, so maintaining a healthy weight is very important. Check your waist circumference by placing a tape measure around your middle while standing. The risk for type 2 diabetes and heart disease increases if the majority of your body fat is concentrated in your waist rather than at your hips. A waist size greater than 35 inches for women and greater than 40 inches for men is associated with elevated risk.

About Metabolic Syndrome

Metabolic syndrome is a name used for a group of risk factors that, if present, increase your risk for having heart disease or other problems such as diabetes. Metabolic syndrome develops for many of the same reasons that prediabetes does. The treatment of metabolic syndrome is the same as for prediabetes. If you have a diagnosis of prediabetes, there may be a good chance that you have metabolic syndrome as well. People who are overweight or obese and physically inactive are more likely to develop metabolic syndrome and insulin resistance. Having excess fat in the abdominal area and a large waist circumference increases the likelihood of insulin resistance.

Insulin resistance is a condition where the body is unable to use its own insulin properly. Insulin, a hormone made by the pancreas, helps the body to use glucose for energy. People with insulin resistance require and may produce more insulin to help glucose get into cells. A consistent overproduction of insulin, coupled with overeating, promotes weight gain. Eventually, the pancreas is no longer able to keep up with insulin demand, and blood glucose begins to rise to the diabetic range. Family history and older age are other possible factors for metabolic syndrome. Obviously, genetics and age cannot be controlled; however, weight, blood fats (blood lipids), blood pressure, and blood glucose are factors that you can have influence over.

Metabolic Syndrome Alert

The conditions that make up metabolic syndrome include: large waist circumference (more than 35 inches in women and 40 inches in men), blood pressure higher than 130/85 mmHg (millimeters of mercury), elevated triglyceride level and a low level of HDL cholesterol, and insulin resistance.

Getting Help: Choosing the Right Doctor

Once you have a confirmed diagnosis, it's time for you to take a step back and decide who will be your partner in managing your prediabetes. If you have a doctor who communicates well, listens to your thoughts and concerns, and seems up to speed on current developments in prediabetes care, you may decide to stay with him or her. However, if your doctor-patient relationship is more on the dysfunctional side, it may be time for you to shop around for someone new. Here are a few questions to consider:

- Does your physician provide cutting-edge care? Is he or she current on the latest clinical studies, new products, and treatment guidelines?
- Is your doctor willing to listen and learn? Does he or she let you voice questions and concerns and give you a chance to ask follow-up questions?
- Is he or she reasonably available? How does he or she handle daytime and after-hours phone calls from patients? Does he or she return calls in a timely manner?
- Does he or she treat the person, not just the disease? Does his or her treatment philosophy reflect a good understanding of the social and emotional impact of prediabetes/diabetes? Does he or she ask questions about your lifestyle to make sure your treatment plan is working?
- What's her bedside manner like? Is he or she abrupt with her staff? Does she brush off patient questions? Do you want a person who isn't nice to be your treatment partner for the lifelong commitment of prediabetes management?
- Does he or she tell it like it is? Having a doctor who explains tests and treatment decisions is essential. He or she should be able to communicate with you frankly and in terms you can understand.

Remember, your doctor is only one member of your healthcare team, albeit an important one. He or she should communicate well with other members of the team as well as with you—sharing information and getting consultation on treatment decisions when appropriate (for instance, working with a neonatologist or ob-gyn to discuss pregnancy issues).

Communication Is Key

Exactly what defines good communication? It's talking with each other rather than at each other—listening instead of just hearing, and explaining rather than commanding. If you ask your doctor why he has ordered a certain test, he should be able to explain his decisions to you in nontechnical language. And if your doctor has questions about your self-care, you should be forthright and honest so he can provide you with the best care possible. The following suggestions may help you improve communication between you and your doctor:

- Think about the symptom(s), questions, and treatment issues you want to discuss in advance. Bring notes if necessary.
- Bring your medications (in their original bottles) with you for doctor visits. This should include herbs and supplements—your doctor should know what you're taking because some supplements may interact with other medications or may be inappropriate for prediabetes patients.
- Treat your doctor as you would like to be treated—respectfully and candidly.
- Bring someone else along to join you after the examination to hear what the doctor recommends.
- If you have been prescribed any medications for prediabetes or other conditions, take your pills as prescribed; if you are not taking your pills, let your doctor know.
- Don't be a "no-show" for appointments, and let the scheduler know exactly what the purpose of the visit is so that she can book your appointment for an appropriate length of time.

Remember, if you don't understand what your doctor is telling you then ask questions. Even after you leave your appointment, don't hesitate to pick up the phone and ask follow-up questions. It's important that you fully comprehend how you are supposed to be treating your prediabetes.

See a General Practitioner after Diagnosis

As long as your doctor has experience treating prediabetes, stays up-to-date on the latest in prediabetes care, is a good partner in your treatment, and communicates well, it really doesn't matter what initials follow her name.

Your Doctor Is Just One Piece of the Healthcare Team Puzzle

Keep in mind that diabetes is a systemic disease that has the potential to affect every part of your body, so preventive care for your prediabetes by a team of trained experts is essential. In addition to your primary care doctor and depending on your medical history, other conditions, and risk factors, you may need to see other specialists. Your primary care physician may be able to provide initial screening for prediabetes-related prevention, but he or she may also refer you to another doctor who has specialized training in a given area of concern or need for screening. Ophthalmologists, mental health providers, nephrologists (doctors who treat diseases related to the kidneys), and podiatrists are just a few of the other care providers who can help you stay healthy and avoid complications.

Food-Savvy RDs

In addition to medical screening and care, dietary management is one of the cornerstones of prediabetes management. A registered dietitian (RD) or a nutritionist who works with patients with prediabetes/diabetes is an essential member of your care team. An RD can teach you concepts like understanding carbohydrates and can explain how certain foods affect blood sugar levels. These professionals can also help you achieve any weight loss goals. Most importantly, your dietitian can also work with you one-on-one to design a meal plan that fits your particular lifestyle. For example, if you're a vegetarian, it will do you little good to get a menu that features fish and meat. Or if, for example, you have a job that keeps you out on the road a great deal of the time, you need someone who can help you make healthy choices outside of your kitchen. Consulting an RD allows you to develop menus that are based in reality. If your diet is practical, then you're more likely to stick to it in the long term.

Dealing with Your Diagnosis

Is your head spinning yet? With all the information thrown at you, through reading, classes, medical appointments, and by well-meaning friends and relatives (who quite frequently spread misinformation rather than fact), feeling overwhelmed is completely normal. Take a deep breath and remember three things:

1. You aren't in this alone—your healthcare team is there to help.
2. You don't have to learn it all at once—control involves some trial and error.
3. Reinventing the wheel is not necessary—others have gone before you, and you'll get through the physical and emotional demands much easier if you join a support group and draw on their wisdom.

It is important to remember that while the information in this book may be extremely helpful, these are general recommendations only, so you will need to work with your doctor to determine the blood sugar and other treatment/outcome goals that are right for you and your particular health picture. And remember, while there are many standardized guidelines and targets in prediabetes care, nearly everything about the condition varies by individual. A food that sends one person's blood sugar off the charts may cause barely a ripple for another.

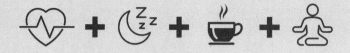

Chapter 2

Know Your Risk, the Symptoms, and Your Treatment Options

NOW THAT YOU have a clear understanding of what prediabetes is and how it is diagnosed, it is important for you to evaluate if you or your family are at risk. You should also become familiar with the signs and symptoms of the condition and how it is treated. These are the first few steps to take before you can develop an action plan to prevent or manage prediabetes as well as prevent the progression to type 2 diabetes.

Prediabetes: Are You at Risk?

An estimated 84.1 million Americans age eighteen and older have prediabetes; worldwide, that number is an estimated 280 million individuals. Many of these people are unaware of their condition. There are a number of known risk factors for both prediabetes and type 2 diabetes. The ADA recommends assessment of risk factors and screening of asymptomatic adults for prediabetes and diabetes. According to their 2018 *Standards of Medical Care* you should be tested for prediabetes/diabetes if you meet the following criteria:

- Adults of any age who are overweight or obese (BMI greater than/ equal to 25, or greater than/equal to 23 in Asian adults) who have one or more of the following risk factors:

  - Belonging to one of the following minority groups: African Americans, Native Americans, Hispanic Americans/Latinos, and Asian Americans/Pacific Islanders
  - Family history of diabetes (especially a first-degree relative)
  - High blood pressure (consistent reading of 140/90 mmHg or higher)
  - Low HDL, or "good," cholesterol (less than 35 mg/dl, or 0.9 mmol/L) and high triglycerides (higher than 250 mg/dl)
  - History of cardiovascular disease
  - Other clinical conditions associated with insulin resistance (severe obesity, acanthosis nigricans)
  - History of polycystic ovary syndrome (PCOS)
  - Physical inactivity

- Patients with a previous hemoglobin A1C test result of 5.7 percent or higher
- Women with gestational diabetes
- Adults age forty-five or over

If results are normal, testing should be repeated at least every three years and sooner if more risk factors are present. Risk factors are used to determine your increased susceptibility to the condition. The more risk factors present in your profile, the greater the risk for developing prediabetes or diabetes. Let's take a look at these risk factors and others in more detail:

Centers for Disease Control and Prevention Statistics

According to the Centers for Disease Control and Prevention (CDC), prediabetes affects about 34 percent of adults eighteen years old and older. About half of adults age sixty-five and older have prediabetes.

Age and Ethnicity

According to the CDC, well over half of all cases of type 2 diabetes occur in people over age fifty, and nearly eleven million Americans age sixty-five and older suffer from the disease. As mentioned previously, individuals older than age forty-five should be tested for diabetes and retested every three years thereafter if the initial test is normal. If you have additional risk factors for type 2 diabetes, you may require more frequent screening—talk to your doctor about your particular screening needs.

Certain ethnic groups and minorities also have an increased risk of developing type 2 diabetes, including the following:

- African Americans
- Asian Americans
- Hispanics
- Pacific Islanders
- Native Americans

Family History

Heredity plays a large part in the development of type 2 diabetes. If you have a first-degree relative with type 2 diabetes, your chances of developing the disease double. There is a concordance rate of up to 90 percent among identical twins with type 2, meaning that in up to 90 percent of cases in which one twin has the disease, the other one develops it as well.

The good news for those with diabetes in their families is that environmental factors such as your activity levels, health habits, and diet play a large role in whether or not you will develop type 2 diabetes. Large-scale studies such as the Diabetes Prevention Program (DPP) have proven that prevention is often possible through eating well, exercise, and other moderate lifestyle changes. Adults in the DPP cut their risk of getting type 2 by over half if they add thirty minutes of exercise five days a week and change their diet, showing that in some cases healthy living can overcome genetics.

Hypertension and Cholesterol Levels and/or History of Cardiovascular Disease

Hypertension, or blood pressure of 140/90 mmHg or higher, is a known risk factor for the development of type 2 diabetes and is also a frequent coexisting condition of the disease. A large-scale study of over 12,000 patients published in *The New England Journal of Medicine* found that people with diagnosed hypertension were two and a half times more likely to develop type 2 diabetes than those individuals with normal blood pressure levels.

CVD and Diabetes

Of those people sixty-five or older with diabetes, at least 68 percent die from some form of heart disease; 16 percent die of stroke. Adults with diabetes are two to four times more likely to die from heart disease than adults who do not have diabetes.

In addition, that study and others have shown a correlation between beta blockers, a medication used to treat high blood pressure, and an increased risk of type 2 diabetes. Triglyceride levels over 250 mg/dl and/or levels of HDL ("good cholesterol") under 35 mg/dl put you at an increased risk for type 2 diabetes. HDL acts as a lubricant for the circulatory system, moving the other lipids (triglycerides and LDL cholesterol) through the blood vessels and into the liver for metabolism. HDL helps to prevent the buildup of fatty plaque that can otherwise clog the arteries, resulting in atherosclerosis and, consequently, high blood pressure.

Elevated triglycerides are also associated with an increased risk of heart disease. There is also a strong relationship between diabetes and cardiovascular disease (CVD) because diabetics often have conditions that predispose them to develop CVD, such as hypertension, abnormal cholesterol, and obesity.

Gestational Diabetes and Perinatal Risk Factors

Women who had gestational diabetes mellitus (GDM) during their pregnancy are at an increased risk of developing type 2 diabetes. Five to 10 percent of women with GDM will have type 2 diabetes after labor and delivery. And women with a history of GDM have a 40–60 percent chance of developing type 2 diabetes within five to ten years postpartum, with a 70 percent risk thereafter. Giving birth to a baby weighing over 9 pounds is also considered a risk factor for later development of type 2 diabetes. Several studies have linked high birth weights (over 4,000 grams, or 8.8 pounds) to type 2 diabetes.

Follow-Up Screenings

Women who have a history of gestational diabetes should be vigilant about regular testing for diabetes (once every three years if glucose levels are normal postpartum, annually if they are not).

Risks Associated with Weight and BMI

Obesity rates have been on a steady rise over the past few decades. The CDC estimates that over 36 percent of US adults are obese. In addition, a growing number of children and adolescents are living with weight issues. According to the 2009–2010 National Health and Nutrition Examination Survey (NHANES), more than 18 percent of adolescents over age twelve, 18 percent of six- to eleven-year-olds, and 12 percent of children between the ages of two and five are considered overweight. For children and adults alike, being overweight or obese is a primary risk factor for developing prediabetes and type 2 diabetes. The US Department of Health and Human Services (HHS) reports that more than 80 percent of people with type 2 diabetes are clinically overweight.

Leptin and Leptin Resistance

Leptin is a hormone in fat cells that helps to metabolize fatty acids, and it has provided an important clue to the relationship between obesity and type 2 diabetes. Discovered by Rockefeller University researchers in 1995, leptin (after the Greek *leptos*, meaning "thin") plays a part in sending a satiety—or "all full"—signal to the brain to stop eating when body fat increases, and an "empty" signal when body fat is insufficient. It appears that a type of leptin resistance may lead to a situation in which fatty acids are deposited instead of metabolized, leading to eventual insulin resistance. Leptin may also play a role in signaling the liver to release stored glucose.

Overweight/Obesity and Insulin Resistance

Too much fat makes it difficult for the body to use its own insulin to process blood glucose and bring it down to normal circulating levels. The specifics are as follows:

- Overweight people have fewer available insulin receptors. When compared to muscle cells, fat cells have fewer insulin receptors where the insulin binds with the cell and "unlocks" it to process glucose into energy.

- More fat requires more insulin. The pancreas starts producing larger and larger quantities of insulin in order to "feed" body mass, and consequently insulin resistance turns into a vicious circle.

- Excess blood sugar must be stored as fat, and excess fat promotes further insulin resistance. Fat cells release free fatty acids (FFAs). During lipolysis (the breakdown of fat within cells), free fatty acids are released into the bloodstream, interfering with glucose metabolism. Abdominal fat appears to release higher levels of FFAs.

Your Personal BMI

Obesity and body fat are measured by body mass index (BMI)—a number that expresses weight in relationship to your height and is a reliable indicator of overall body fat. People with a BMI of 25 to 29.9 are considered overweight; those with a BMI of 30 or over are obese. You should aim for a BMI of 18.5 to 24.9, which is considered normal. BMI is calculated differently for children and for young adults ages two to nineteen. A charting system called BMI-for-age compares each child's weight in relation to other children of the same age and gender on a growth chart in terms of percentiles. For example, a girl in the thirteenth percentile would weigh the same or more than 13 percent of girls the same age. A healthy BMI for children is from the fifth to less than the eighty-fifth percentile. Growth charts used for assessing pediatric BMI-for-age are based on NHANES data and are generated by the CDC. A BMI-for-age that is at the ninety-fifth percentile or higher is considered obese, while the eighty-fifth to less than the ninety-fifth percentile is overweight.

BMI	19	20	21	22	23	24	25	26	27	28	29	30	31	32	33	34	35	36	37	38	39
Height (inches)	Body weight (pounds)																				
58	91	96	100	105	110	115	119	124	129	134	138	143	148	153	158	162	167	172	177	181	186
59	94	99	104	109	114	119	124	128	133	138	143	148	153	158	163	168	173	178	183	188	193
60	97	102	107	112	118	123	128	133	138	143	148	153	158	163	168	174	179	184	189	194	199
61	100	106	111	116	122	127	132	137	143	148	153	158	164	169	174	180	185	190	195	201	206
62	104	109	115	120	126	131	136	142	147	153	158	164	169	175	180	186	191	196	202	207	213
63	107	113	118	124	130	135	141	146	152	158	163	169	175	180	186	191	197	203	208	214	220
64	110	116	122	128	134	140	145	151	157	163	169	174	180	186	192	197	204	209	215	221	227
65	114	120	126	132	138	144	150	156	162	168	174	180	186	192	198	204	210	216	222	228	234
66	118	124	130	136	142	148	155	161	167	173	179	186	192	198	204	210	216	223	229	235	241
67	121	127	134	140	146	153	159	166	172	178	185	191	198	204	211	217	223	230	236	242	249
68	125	131	138	144	151	158	164	171	177	184	190	197	203	210	216	223	230	236	243	249	256
69	128	135	142	149	155	162	169	176	182	189	196	203	209	216	223	230	236	243	250	257	263
70	132	139	146	153	160	167	174	181	188	195	202	209	216	222	229	236	243	250	257	264	271
71	136	143	150	157	165	172	179	186	193	200	208	215	222	229	236	243	250	257	265	272	279
72	140	147	154	162	169	177	184	191	199	206	213	221	228	235	242	250	258	265	272	279	287
73	144	151	159	166	174	182	189	197	204	212	219	227	235	242	250	257	265	272	280	288	295
74	148	155	163	171	179	186	194	202	210	218	225	233	241	249	256	264	272	280	287	295	303
75	152	160	168	176	184	192	200	208	216	224	232	240	248	256	264	272	279	287	295	303	311
76	156	164	172	180	189	197	205	213	221	230	238	246	254	263	271	279	287	295	304	312	320

Normal   Overweight   Obese

Body mass index (BMI) table

Body Shape

Having an apple-shaped body, with excess pounds packed in the midsection rather than the hips, is another hallmark of insulin resistance. In fact, the National Institutes of Health recommends that waist circumference be used as a screening tool for evaluating the risk of heart disease and type 2 diabetes.

CLASSIFICATION OF OVERWEIGHT AND OBESITY BY BMI, WAIST CIRCUMFERENCE, AND ASSOCIATED RISK OF TYPE 2 DIABETES, HYPERTENSION, AND CARDIOVASCULAR DISEASE		
Disease Risk Relative to Normal Weight and Waist Circumference		
	BMI (kg/m2)	≤102 cm. (≤40 in.) for men; ≤88 cm. (≤35 in.) for women	>102 cm. (>40 in.) for men; >88 cm. (>35 in.) for women
Underweight	<18.5	no increased risk	no increased risk
Normal	18.5–24.9	no increased risk	no increased risk
Overweight	25.0–29.9	increased	high
Obesity	30.0–34.9	high	very high
Obesity	35.0–39.9	very high	very high

Polycystic Ovary Syndrome and Prediabetes

Polycystic ovary syndrome (PCOS) affects approximately 5–10 percent of women in the US. PCOS is defined as a grouping of reproductive health problems characterized by polycystic ("many cysts") ovaries, irregular menstrual cycles, infertility, and obesity. It is the most common cause of irregular menstrual cycles and infertility. Most women with PCOS have insulin resistance and hyperinsulinism. Hyperinsulinism means that high amounts of insulin are routinely produced to combat the insulin resistance. Like metabolic syndrome, an overproduction of insulin triggers a cycle of easy weight gain. Some women with PCOS also have metabolic syndrome and may have other symptoms such as acanthosis nigricans (dark skin patches), acne, facial hair, or loss of scalp hair. A woman with PCOS can go on to develop prediabetes or type 2 diabetes. Other conditions associated with PCOS may include obstructive sleep apnea, depression, or hypothyroidism.

Other Risk Factors

Other risk factors that are possibly related to weight and prediabetes/diabetes are an inactive lifestyle and inadequate sleep. Exercise, even at a moderate level, reduces blood glucose levels and helps control weight. People who lead sedentary lifestyles, exercising fewer than three times a week, are more likely to develop type 2 diabetes than those who are more active.

There is also a possibility that too little or too much sleep may play a role in developing diabetes. A recent review of several studies looking at sleep's effect showed that lowest risk of type 2 diabetes was found in those obtaining 7–8 hours a night and that any less or more may increase risk. Possible mechanisms for a relationship to short sleep duration may be increased food intake, disturbances in hormones, metabolism, glucose tolerance, and insulin sensitivity, whereas longer sleep duration may be associated with lower physical activity and higher inflammation in the body. More research needs to be done to reach better and more specific conclusions regarding this topic.

It is important to keep in mind that the biggest indicator for your risk of type 2 diabetes is the diagnosed presence of prediabetes. But because the vast majority of people with prediabetes remain undiagnosed, assessing the presence of the other common risk factors for type 2 diabetes is important.

Know Your Risk *and* the Symptoms

In addition to knowing the risk factors for developing prediabetes/diabetes, it is also important to be familiar with the symptoms that may indicate you have it. Symptoms associated with prediabetes can be nonexistent or indistinguishable from other causes. Early symptoms of prediabetes are so common, in fact, that many people barely notice them at all or think that what they are feeling is "normal."

The symptoms can be vague and rarely interfere with daily activities. However, sometimes the red flags associated with type 2 diabetes begin to appear, such as:

- Increased thirst
- Frequent urination
- Fatigue that doesn't improve with more sleep
- Blurred vision that may come and go
- Acanthosis nigricans (darkening of the skin in certain areas, such as the neck, armpits, elbows, knees, or knuckles)

You may have several symptoms before you begin to realize that things are not quite right.

Prediabetes in Special Populations: Pregnancy and Children

Prediabetes does not affect only adults. It can happen in pregnant women and in children. The sections that follow help explain risk factors, screening, and diagnosis of prediabetes during pregnancy and in children.

Pregnancy and Prediabetes

Pregnancy is a time of life when most women are highly motivated to take very good care of themselves. They do this because they want the best possible outcome for their baby. For a woman with either prediabetes or gestational diabetes, good self-care is especially important and necessary to ensure a good outcome. Though there are differences between prediabetes and gestational diabetes, keep in mind that there is a definite connection between the two as well.

The diagnostic criteria for prediabetes usually starts with a fasting blood glucose between 100–125 mg/dl on more than one occasion. If a woman has prediabetes at the onset of her pregnancy, her risk for developing gestational diabetes is increased. And conversely, women who have a history of GDM during their pregnancy are at an increased risk of developing prediabetes or type 2 diabetes after delivery and in the future.

Gestational Diabetes

Somewhere between 2–10 percent of all pregnant women develop gestational diabetes. It is more common in women who are older or overweight at the onset of their pregnancy, or if they had gestational diabetes in a prior pregnancy. Gestational diabetes occurs when certain hormones from the placenta interfere with the normal action of the woman's insulin. Hormonal interference creates insulin resistance, and the woman's ability to use her own insulin to regulate blood sugar is greatly reduced. The pancreas, which produces insulin, cannot produce enough insulin to correct the insulin resistance, and high blood sugar levels are the result. All pregnant women are screened for gestational diabetes between twenty-four and twenty-eight weeks of the pregnancy. This is generally the time when gestational diabetes becomes evident. Women with glucose abnormalities such as prediabetes or a prior history of gestational diabetes may be screened earlier than this.

The screening is done by measuring the mother's blood glucose one hour after she has consumed 50 grams of glucose. A blood glucose of 140 mg/dl or less is considered normal; if it is higher than that, further testing is done. When a second round of testing is performed, 100 grams of glucose are consumed, and the blood glucose is measured at the fasting level and every hour for the next two to three hours. Levels greater than the values that follow are indicative of gestational diabetes:

- Fasting: 92 mg/dl
- One hour: 180 mg/dl
- Two hours: 155 mg/dl
- Three hours: 140 mg/dl

Even under normal conditions, pregnancy is a stressful time for the body. In addition to the normal stresses of pregnancy, having prediabetes makes the risk for gestational diabetes that much greater. If you have prediabetes and are planning to become pregnant, be sure to get your prediabetes under control first. Discuss your plans for starting a family with your doctor and follow recommendations for getting healthier before the pregnancy. It may be a good idea to monitor your blood glucose a few times weekly and have your doctor check your hemoglobin A1c to determine whether your prediabetes is well controlled. If you have been diagnosed with gestational diabetes you will need to work closely with your doctor and likely a registered dietitian to develop an individualized treatment plan that includes lifestyle changes such as diet and exercise.

I'm Pregnant and Have Prediabetes...Now What?

If you are already pregnant and have prediabetes, it does not necessarily mean that you will develop gestational diabetes. Be proactive by improving your lifestyle habits right away. Some of the habits discussed later in this book may be helpful, but you will need to consult with your doctor and a dietitian first and develop an individualized diet and exercise plan that is safe and right for you. Keeping weight gain under control throughout the pregnancy can help minimize your chances of developing gestational diabetes. Follow your doctor's recommendations for the right amount of weight to gain during your pregnancy. Here are recommended guidelines for weight gain based on your weight at the start of the pregnancy:

- Underweight: 28–40 pounds
- Normal weight: 25–35 pounds
- Overweight: 15–25 pounds
- Obese: 11–20 pounds

After Delivery

In most cases, in women who had gestational diabetes, it goes away after the baby is born. This is because the mother no longer has the hormones that interfered with insulin and raised her blood glucose. But again, women with a gestational diabetes history may be predisposed to prediabetes/type 2 diabetes at a later time in life.

The woman with prediabetes prior to or during her pregnancy may or may not have prediabetes afterward. The outcome in this situation is dependent upon certain variables such as amount of weight gain, diet, exercise, or level of glucose control during the pregnancy.

Whether you had to manage prediabetes or gestational diabetes during pregnancy, your decision to prevent type 2 diabetes requires a certain amount of vigilance after you have your baby. Following the healthy habits mentioned later in this book will be a great start. By staying on course with a healthy lifestyle, you will be taking the steps within your control to prevent type 2 diabetes in the future.

Children and Teens with Prediabetes

With the medical advances over the decades, a gradual increase in the human life span has occurred for each successive generation. Now this trend may change, and for the first time in many years, today's children could have health issues or chronic disease at a much earlier age compared to their parents or grandparents. Earlier onset of chronic disease could mean a decline in the life expectancies of the younger generation. The increased incidence of obesity and prediabetes in our children plays a major role in this unfortunate development.

Thirty years ago, it was uncommon to see a child with prediabetes/diabetes. Today healthcare practitioners not only see children and adolescents with prediabetes; they also diagnose and treat type 2 diabetes in this same population. Type 2 diabetes was once regarded as an adult-onset form of diabetes, not a form of diabetes that affected children or adolescents. According to data from the National Diabetes Fact Sheet 2007, there were approximately two million adolescents (or one in six overweight adolescents) with prediabetes.

Children and teens are more at risk for prediabetes or diabetes if:

- They are overweight or obese (a BMI greater than the eighty-fifth percentile for age and sex, a weight for height greater than the eighty-fifth percentile, or a weight greater than 120 percent of ideal for height)
- They have a parent, sibling, or other close relative with type 2 diabetes
- They do not get enough physical activity
- They are American Indian, African American, Asian American, or Hispanic/Latino

Although it is not possible to change your genetic or family background, maintaining a healthy weight and staying active are two areas that you and your child have control of. It is much easier to correct a small problem before it becomes a big problem. If your child is gaining extra weight, take steps to reverse the situation as soon as possible. Even if your child displays no signs of prediabetes, a healthy weight and adequate activity are vitally important in the prevention of this condition.

The Role of BMI in Children

For many years doctors relied on height and weight measurements to assess a child's growth pattern. Height and weight are usually reviewed during the annual health checkup. Another way to determine whether a child is at a healthy weight is to calculate his or her body mass index (BMI). BMI is a calculation that uses height and weight to estimate how much body fat a person has. The BMI calculation for children is not interpreted in the same way as normal BMI ranges for adults. Although the mathematical method used to determine the BMI is the same, a child's BMI is compared to typical values for other children of the same age and gender. For children ages two through nineteen, a BMI that is less than the fifth percentile is considered underweight, and a BMI above the ninety-fifth percentile is considered obese. A BMI between the eighty-fifth and ninety-fifth percentile is classified as overweight.

Check Your Child's BMI and BMI Percentile

You can ask your doctor to determine this or check it on your own, using the KidsHealth BMI Calculator found at this website: https:// kidshealth.org/en/parents/bmi-charts.html. To use this calculator, you will need to enter height, weight, age, and gender.

If your child's BMI indicates an overweight status, keep in mind that he or she is still growing. In some cases, an overweight child may grow out of the overweight category as he gets taller and older. Because of growth, it is important to check your child's BMI routinely, to see whether it has improved or gotten worse. When children or teens remain in the overweight or obese category, there should be screening for prediabetes and diabetes. Screening is especially important when additional risk factors such as family history of diabetes or ethnic specificity are present.

The laboratory tests to screen children and teens for prediabetes or diabetes are the same as those used for adults. A fasting blood glucose (after an overnight fast) should be under 100 mg/dl. Some doctors prefer to use the glucose challenge when screening children. Based on the child's body weight, a specific number of grams of glucose are consumed, and the blood glucose is checked two hours later. A healthy child will have a result of less than 140 mg/dl after two hours. A blood sugar level from 140 to

199 mg/dl is considered prediabetes, and a blood sugar level of 200 mg/dl or higher indicates type 2 diabetes. If the hemoglobin A1c test is used, a result of 5.7–6.4 percent is indicative of prediabetes.

What to Do If Your Child Has Prediabetes

As upsetting as the news may be, your child's diagnosis of prediabetes is very treatable and, with the right plan in place, reversible. Put your child's mind at ease by letting him know that you are going to be there to help. It is important for your child to understand that certain changes in eating and exercise habits are necessary to prevent future health problems. At the same time, you need to present this information in a way so that your child does not become fearful or excessively worried about his condition.

To have success with lifestyle improvements, change really has to become a family affair. In other words, you and other family members must be supportive and participate in the lifestyle changes that need to take place. Don't expect your child or teen to "go it alone," while others in the household continue to have poor eating or lifestyle habits. If your child feels as though she has been singled out, you will very likely meet with resistance. Many of the healthy habits mentioned in this book will be helpful to use as a family, but always consult with your child's physician and dietitian first before making any changes.

It is important to get your child actively engaged and involved in the process of change. She will be more likely to "buy in" to new changes when she is involved in some of the decision-making and not just told what to do. For example, let your child decide what healthy after-school snack she would like to eat, instead of selecting items for her. Although grocery shopping takes more time with children present, it is worthwhile to take your child along from time to time. Shopping trips can help your child see and learn about different food options, as well as provide an opportunity to choose healthy foods. As a parent, your most important job is to set a good example, and having a healthy lifestyle is no exception. Early on, children learn by example and copy their parents' behavior. For example, parents who don't eat vegetables can hardly expect their child to start eating them willingly on their own! Model healthy lifestyle and eating habits listed in this book yourself, and you will have a much better chance of getting your child to follow your good example.

Some Things to Keep in Mind with Children

By now you understand the importance of helping your child start a healthy eating and exercise program sooner rather than later. Most of us (your child included) have established eating habits that may be hard to break. Working little by little on ways to eat healthier takes time and patience. The same goes for taking on more activity or exercise. A child who prefers passive activities such as watching television will need time to get used to getting physical activity every day. Old habits are hard to break and without daily practice of new habits, it's easy to get off track or revert to old behavior. Success usually comes by starting with small changes and mastering a new behavior before taking on more challenges. One or two positive changes at a time are realistic and prevent your child from becoming overwhelmed. Do not get discouraged if your child or teen does not immediately change all of his poor health habits. Even adults struggle with lifestyle change and have to try over and over again. Your job is to encourage your child to keep trying.

Ultimately, children and teens want to be accepted by their peers. At some level they understand that being overweight or having health problems can make it more difficult to develop friendships, play in sports, or participate in social activities. Healthy habits will help your child gain more confidence and control over his or her own well-being, and this can have a positive effect on other areas of your child's life.

Treatment Approaches

Multiple long-term, large-scale studies have shown that the best way to prevent the progression from prediabetes to diabetes in those at risk is through intensive changes in lifestyle and maintaining these changes over time. A good diet, regular activity, and losing weight (for those who are overweight or obese) are still considered the best and first-line approach.

The majority of this book will be dedicated to discussing healthy habits centered on these core principles and other important lifestyle factors that can promote diabetes prevention and longevity. But you may be wondering if there are other treatments, medications even, that can be used to treat or prevent prediabetes, so first it is important to touch on the latest research and developments in the realm of prediabetes care.

Medications for Prediabetes?

Currently there are no FDA-approved medications for treating prediabetes, so lifestyle changes are most commonly recommended. However, the oral medication metformin has been studied in recent years for its potential to tame prediabetes and prevent its progression. Metformin belongs to a class of drugs called biguanides and has been used for many years as a first-line agent to treat diabetes. It helps lower blood glucose levels by preventing the liver from releasing excess glucose and by helping the muscle and fat cells become more sensitive to the body's available insulin.

The Diabetes Prevention Program (DPP) was a very large multicenter trial that compared the use of metformin versus lifestyle intervention to see if either was superior in preventing or at least delaying the onset of diabetes in subjects who were at high risk. The study showed that lifestyle intervention was the most effective approach and decreased the incidence of type 2 diabetes by 58 percent compared with 31 percent in the metformin-treated group. Subsequent studies have also demonstrated the important benefit of lifestyle intervention in significantly reducing risk. Even though changes in lifestyle are generally recommended first, it has been determined through further analysis that some particular groups may benefit from metformin in addition to lifestyle changes so much so that more recent American Diabetes Association *Standards of Medical Care in Diabetes* state that metformin therapy for prevention of type 2 diabetes should be considered to treat those with prediabetes whose BMI is more than 35 kg/m2, persons younger than sixty years old, and women with a history of gestational diabetes mellitus as well as women diagnosed with PCOS.

Watch Vitamin B_{12} Blood Levels

While metformin is one the longest-used oral medications for diabetes and has a good safety profile, long-term use of it can lead to vitamin B_{12} deficiency. Blood levels of vitamin B_{12} should be measured at regular intervals by those taking the medication, especially those with a history of anemia or nerve damage.

Other oral and injectable diabetes medicines as well as weight loss medicines have shown some promise in studies to help with prediabetes, yet metformin is the most well studied to date, and none of these have been approved specifically to treat the condition. For now, lifestyle changes are still considered the safest, lowest in cost, and often most effective first option to try.

Your Action Plan to Tackle Prediabetes

By now you understand the potential consequences of untreated prediabetes. It is important to develop an action plan to manage and, with hard work on your part, reverse it. Your action plan will help you make lifestyle changes gradually that you will implement on a day-to-day basis. Halting the progression of prediabetes is extremely important and necessary to restore good health. With prediabetes, there is still a chance for you to reverse the progression and prevent the onset of type 2 diabetes. Even if you develop diabetes at a later time, slowing down the progression will result in fewer complications. If you don't take action, progression to full-blown type 2 diabetes is a likely possibility.

There are multiple important components to your action plan based on healthy habits that will be outlined in the remaining chapters:

- Make dietary changes: eat for better blood sugar control and good health
- Engage in regular activity: exercise for better blood sugar control and good health
- Get to a healthy weight (if you are overweight or obese); lose weight for better blood sugar control and good health
- Reduce stress, sleep more, and love more: create a positive lifestyle for better blood sugar control and good health
- Correct bad habits that are setting you back: replace them with new habits that promote better blood sugar control and good health

Before tackling the action plan and the habits that support it, first it is important to understand what a habit really is, how habits are formed, and how behavior change can come about, as well as the significance of setting the right types of goals to create habits for a healthy lifestyle that will last.

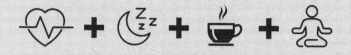

Chapter 3

Important Tools for Lasting Behavioral and Health Change

BEHAVIOR HAS A powerful influence on health, so much so that even the most detailed and comprehensive lifestyle plan is destined to fail unless it includes a sound behavior modification component. A large part of behavioral change centers on your habits. Developing and focusing on the right kind of habits empowers you to turn your best intentions and the knowledge you have acquired about ways to change your lifestyle (such as diet and exercise) into a reality. Learning more about habits, understanding the science behind them, and uncovering ways to develop healthy positive habits are all key to lasting lifestyle changes.

What Is a Habit?

Habits are, undoubtedly, a major part of our everyday routine. From the time you get up in the morning until the evening when your head hits the pillow to go to sleep, your day is filled with countless actions and choices, almost half of which may be habits. In fact, the life of humans (and other living creatures) has been characterized largely as a "bundle of habits" by William James, a famous Harvard psychologist and philosopher who led some of the earliest investigations about the psychology and neurology behind habits through his work in the late 1800s. Since then countless studies have been conducted to research how habits are formed and maintained, by looking at brain activity and behaviors, and the results have been fascinating.

"Creature of Habit": Where Did That Phrase Come From?

No exact source can be pinpointed for the common phrase "creature of habit," yet variations of it were created and published by early prominent psychologists of the late 1800s. Examples include: "Man is largely a creature of habit, and many of his activities are more or less automatic reflexes from the stimuli of his environment" by G. Stanley Hall and "When we look at living creatures from an outward point of view, one of the first things that strikes us is that they are bundles of habits" from William James.

While the precise definition of habit has been debated and is described differently in a variety of psychological and neurological contexts, the most common definition of habit seems to center around the following concept: habits are automatic behavioral responses to environmental cues or triggers. The part of the brain called the basal ganglia plays a large role in habit development. The basal ganglia consists of clusters of neurons called nuclei, which are located in the base of the forebrain (the largest part of the brain). This group of neurons is thought to be responsible for the selection of actions that lead to habit formation.

How Do Habits Form?

There are countless theories as to how habits are learned and created, how they develop, and why they persist. One of the most common explanations of habit formation is offered by Ann Graybiel, a PhD and professor who has conducted extensive research in the area of habits and the basal ganglia. Her explanation involves the following sequence of events:

- First, you acquire a habit by experience(s) that leads to creation and organization of neuron connections in your brain (also referred to as experience-dependent plasticity).
- Second, you repeat the habit behavior over time; do it enough, and it can become fixed.
- Third, the habit is fully acquired, and you now perform it automatically, without requiring direct attention or focus.
- Fourth, the habit becomes a sequence of actions that tends to occur in response to a particular situation or cue.

Essentially, according to this and other similar theories, once habits are learned, repeated, and acquired, they occur automatically. Tasks such as preparing a cup of coffee or brushing your teeth, once you learn them through a series of steps that required significant concentration and time, have been well integrated into your routine. Now you perform them with barely any thought. We rely on habits because they allow us to perform a variety of actions in daily life, often while doing other things, without having to stop and fully concentrate on what we are doing, thus saving time and energy.

Habitual Cues

A cue is an impulse or trigger that leads to a routine, such as a habit. Cues can be external—coming from the environment, or internal—which come from within. Examples of external cues are a location, a time of day, or other people or places; for instance, going to the movies is a cue for the habit of eating popcorn. Internal cues include mood, thinking patterns, and sensations in the body, such as the feeling of hunger making you want to eat.

The Importance of Habits for Good Health

It's no secret that habits are key to health. They can make or break your chances of achieving and maintaining wellness goals such as eating right, staying fit, managing prediabetes and other medical conditions, along with increasing your quality of life and promoting longevity. There is plenty of data showing that bad habits like increased consumption of soft drinks and fast food, as well as low activity levels, are linked to development of chronic diseases such as obesity and diabetes. In contrast, healthy habits such as high consumption of fruits and vegetables, eating more fresh foods, and exercising regularly can provide many health benefits, such as helping achieve a proper weight and lowering the risk of diseases such as cancer and diabetes. Taking a look at your current habits, deciding what needs to be changed, and then learning how to increase positive habits, as well as reduce negative ones, is an important step toward helping you manage your prediabetes and overall health.

Making the Decision to Change

Changing your habits takes time and effort. In order to adopt new habits and get rid of old ones to improve your health, you need to be in the right mind-set and do your best to put yourself in an environment that favors change. Frequent barriers to changing habits and behavior include:

- Not being ready
- Not seeing the needed changes as important
- Not believing in yourself and not able to think that change can happen
- Not having a social support network
- Not having a good plan, knowledge, or tools to help make change happen

Understanding the stages of change and figuring out where you are in the process can help you tremendously in dealing with any potential roadblocks and allow you to make change happen.

How Change Takes Place

There are many theories that address and explain behavior change, but one of the most comprehensive and widely accepted models of behavior change used today is called the transtheoretical model of change, developed by psychologists James Prochaska and Carlo DiClemente in the late 1970s. It helps explain the main stages individuals go through when making a change:

1. Precontemplation: you are not ready to make a change anytime soon.
2. Contemplation: you are thinking about and possibly getting ready to make a change.
3. Preparation: you are now ready to actually make the change and beginning to take steps to change.
4. Action: you are actively making specific changes in behavior through taking action.
5. Maintenance: you have made changes and have been able to sustain them for over six months.

Becoming Familiar with the Change Process

Identifying where you are in the stages of change can help you realize what your current situation is when it comes to making a change in your habits. It will also help you investigate what it may take to move forward. Let's look at an example to illustrate what you might do if you found yourself in any of these particular stages—for instance, if you wanted to make the change to eating fruit instead of candy as your after-dinner snack.

Precontemplation Stage

If you were in the precontemplation stage, you would have no intention of substituting the fruit for the candy. Acknowledging your ambivalence to change and learning or thinking more about the potential benefits of eating the fruit and avoiding the candy—for example, its effects on weight and blood sugar—may be helpful to motivate you to get to the next stage. Seeking the help of a dietitian or behavioral therapist can be useful in this stage to help you discuss your current state and understand the concrete health benefits of changing.

Contemplation Stage

Being in the contemplation stage means you are actually considering making the change to eat the fruit. In this case you may know about the pros and cons of making the change process. You may really crave that candy; it is a nightly ritual that brings feelings of comfort or satisfaction. Focus on the positive aspects of eating fruit, such as cutting calories, sugar, and fat and adding fiber and nutrients. Reinforce any affirming self-motivations ("I can do this, I have made changes in the past!") to stop eating the candy. Again, a health professional who will work with you one-on-one to explore pros and cons and develop ways to overcome resistance can assist you tremendously in this stage.

Preparation Stage

When you reach the preparation stage, you are ready to eat the fruit instead of the candy and are making plans to make this change. Thinking about small, specific, and realistic steps you can take, such as making the commitment to stop buying candy to have in the house, making a list of fruit you enjoy to buy at the store, and ways you can preprepare fruit to have readily available to eat would be great steps to take at this stage. Working with a health professional to help set the right goals can be beneficial at this point if you are having trouble identifying key steps. In addition, letting others know about the change you intend to make so they can support you is important at this stage as well.

Action Stage

Once in the action stage, you have changed your behavior and replaced the candy with fruit after dinner. You will need to focus on repetition and reinforcement of this behavior so it becomes a habit. It's important to focus on your success as a motivator to keep eating the fruit instead of the candy and continuing to enlist the support of others to encourage you with this habit. Make sure no one is tempting you by bringing candy into the house. Acknowledge the challenge of maintaining this healthy habit by planning ahead and developing coping strategies when in high-risk situations—for instance, how you might deal with eating fruit instead of a sugary dessert when you go to a restaurant.

Maintenance Stage

In the maintenance phase you have successfully stopped eating the candy and replaced it with fruit for more than six months. At this point you will work to sustain this change and prevent relapse. You may also want to try finding creative ways to stick to your routine, like trying new fruit and fruit recipes. In addition, you will identify times when you are at risk of relapsing (for instance, during an after-dinner movie). You'll figure out how to deal with these situations to keep to your new lifestyle habit. If you have had a setback, such as indulging in too much candy at a holiday party, you'll deal with it by acknowledging the issue, analyzing what led to the problem, and revisiting how to get back on track and stay there.

Knowing the stages of change can be eye-opening and empowering when you're trying to make changes in your behavior, to develop good habits, and to manage your prediabetes. As well, this knowledge helps you squash the not-so-good habits that are barriers to maintaining a healthy lifestyle. Becoming self-aware, having confidence in yourself, acquiring the knowledge and skills to set goals, and reaching out for support from friends, family members, and healthcare providers are all important things to consider when going through the stages of change.

Help from the Professionals

One of the most common counseling techniques used by health-care professionals today is called motivational interviewing. In contrast to the traditional informational model of counseling that is more prescriptive and based on telling you what to do (which can also include confrontation and "scare tactics"), motivational interviewing takes a different approach. This evidence-based technique centers on the idea that change should come from within you by helping you explore your own mixed or opposed feelings, known as ambivalence. This in turn encourages you to change by partnering with a therapist. When a healthcare professional uses motivational interviewing techniques, she actively listens to you, is empathetic and supportive to your concerns, and encourages you to express your own motivations to change. This strengthens your commitment and your intention to make change actually happen.

Harnessing the Power of Habits

Making the decision to change your habits, namely decreasing the ones that are harmful and increasing or adding those that are beneficial, is a great first step toward managing your prediabetes. But then how do you move forward to take action and change these habits? The topic of habit change and its ability to impact and improve health has been studied for over 100 years. There are a number of strategies based on a variety of research that you can learn to help you change and/or adopt habits for lifestyle change. Think about which of the following tips, tricks, and techniques may be right for you, and remember: trial and error, an open mind, and some patience will be key.

Learn All You Can

You may be curious and want to modify your lifestyle, but you're not sure how. Studies have shown that education can help increase your intention and motivation to change, thus inspiring you to take action. Reading this book is a great start; the following chapters are chock-full of useful ideas and suggestions about ways to add more healthy habits to your routine. In addition, reaching out to a health professional, such as a registered dietitian and/or behavioral therapist to get one-on-one instruction can be another wonderful way to learn more. These professionals can educate and partner with you to jump-start the habit change process.

Pay Attention to Your Cues and Your Actions

As mentioned previously, a cue is an impulse or trigger that leads to a routine, such as a habit. They range from external (part of your environment: a specific location, a time of day, other people or places) to internal (from within yourself: feelings, thinking patterns, and sensations in the body). Charles Duhigg, in his bestseller *The Power of Habit*, suggests that there is an actual "habit loop" we go through when developing and experiencing habits. It all starts with a cue. He describes a three-step process in the brain:

1. Cue: first there is a cue, an initiator, that signals the brain to begin the habit.
2. Routine: then comes a behavioral action that is taken as a result of the cue.
3. Reward: finally there is a benefit that is experienced as a result of the routine, which will reinforce the brain to encode the habit for continued use in the future.

Identifying the cues that trigger your habits is an important beginning step to changing the behavior, namely bad habits.

- Is there a certain time of day or place (like the couch!) when/where you tend to snack?
- Does being with certain people cause you to stay out too late and miss sleep?
- Do certain moods affect your ability to stick to your exercise routine?

Taking note of the cues that lead to some of your habits can help you to become aware of what leads you to engage in certain behaviors so you can try to identify what you are doing wrong as a result and ways you might change that. On the flip side, adding in certain cues to encourage new and positive health habit formation is important too, such as putting a large water bottle on your desk to prompt you to drink more or putting your gym clothes in the car to remind you to go to the gym after work.

In some cases, you may be able to change some of the cues, like avoiding certain environments or people that are bad influences, but it has been suggested that changing the behavior that results from the cue and/or the reward is more realistic and beneficial.

Self-Monitoring Can Help

A great deal of research has shown that keeping food and activity diaries can help promote healthy behavior, and noting specific cues that come before the behavior can be especially useful. A recent study conducted in 2014 showed that participants who kept a cue-monitoring diary found that it helped decrease unhealthy snacking in comparison to those subjects using the control diary who did not focus on recording cues.

In addition to describing the habit loop (cue-routine-reward) that proposes how habits are formed, Duhigg has also suggested a way to transform habits by using the "golden rule of habit change." This involves allowing the cue and the reward to remain the same and just changing the routine that connects them. For example, if you normally go out with your friends (cue) to eat somewhere that is not healthy (routine) mainly to enjoy their companionship (reward), instead you could spend time with friends in an activity not centered around food, like a walk or concert, so you are able to enjoy the reward of their companionship without sabotaging your eating plan. Or if you are normally hungry in the afternoon (cue) and have a cookie (routine) to satisfy yourself (reward), you could change your routine to having a piece of fruit that will still decrease your hunger in a healthier way. Developing a competing routine that is more positive and healthful can help bring about change that is good for you in response to your usual cues. And it will still yield a similar, if not the same, reward.

Rethink Your Rewards

Another strategy that has been proven to be successful with adopting healthy habits is to change the way you reward yourself, namely if what you normally do is working against your attempts to change your lifestyle. If you commonly celebrate successes in life by using food as a reward, then keep the habit of celebrating your accomplishment, but replace the reward with a nonfood treat, such as a new book or a shopping trip with a friend. If you use TV time on the couch to indulge yourself after a long day, instead take a walk with a friend or enroll in a yoga class to relax and recharge. This is another example of reframing and replacing the way you acknowledge yourself, but doing so in a healthier way.

Repeat, Repeat, Repeat...

Research has shown time and time again that the more you repeat a behavioral routine, the more likely it is to become a habit. Use this concept to your advantage. If you know how to eat healthy, exercise, and make other lifestyle changes to manage your prediabetes, then get out there and try it. Do it often and then some! The more times you allow yourself to put your intentions and knowledge into practice via action, the easier it becomes. Repeating healthy behaviors increases skill, motivation, and confidence, which are all key to maintaining long-lasting habits for success. On the other end of the spectrum, realize that the more you go on repeating unhealthy habits, the harder it becomes to break them. "Old habits die hard," they say. The more you repeat something, the more automatic it becomes. Use that principle in your favor, and don't let it work against you.

Let Your Habits Build upon Each Other

If you tie a new healthy habit to an existing one, the potential for change and success multiplies. Some examples are:

- Go to bed early so it will be easier for you to wake up for your regular exercise class
- Grab a piece of fruit after your workout
- Add a big glass of water before your healthy meal or talk about your stressors with a friend while walking instead of sitting at the local coffee shop

Find opportunities to multitask in a good way to let your healthy habits build upon each other. This will increase motivation and expand your network of healthy habits.

Setting Yourself Up for Success

Studies show that you are more likely to be successful with changing your behavior and sticking with a healthy habit if you are not only ready to change but you also believe in yourself and have support. Gaining knowledge and skills by educating yourself and using your resources is important in creating the lifestyle habits you need to manage your prediabetes and health. As you continue to learn and practice your habits, things will get easier and you will be able to take on new challenges and build on past successes. You want to surround yourself with people who will elevate you to help you reach your goals and minimize interactions with those who do not have your best interests in mind and only want to encourage old routines or bad habits.

Positive communication is of the utmost importance. If you are having trouble getting started, are lacking confidence in your abilities, or require more education to achieve your goals, reach out to your medical team, family, and friends to get the help and support you need to start. It will make a big difference in the beginning and throughout your journey of changing and maintaining your lifestyle habits.

Plan to Deal with Challenges and Setbacks

When trying to change your habits and add new, positive ones, realize that this is a process and that challenges and setbacks can happen. Some challenges you can plan for in advance, and others may present themselves out of the blue, and you will have to do your best to work to overcome them. Always remember the value of keeping a positive attitude. Stress and negative thoughts are draining and have the potential to derail your efforts. They can make it difficult to maintain your healthy habits and can even lead to new bad habits or allow you relapse to previous undesirable ones, so it is important for you to get a handle on them. Beware of the "all-or-nothing" attitude that can set you up for failure. If you make a mistake, realize that you are human, give yourself some credit, and try to learn from it. Developing healthy coping techniques is key to having the upper hand when going through challenging times. If you need help with working on stress management and coping techniques, as well as goal setting, working with a healthcare professional may be a good idea for you to be able to learn and succeed.

Goals: Important Counterparts of Healthy Habits

Setting goals is important to the process of behavior change and developing the right kind of habits. Goals can help influence habit formation by motivating you to start a habit, repeat it, and maintain it. There are several things to keep in mind when setting goals so that that you can set yourself up for attainable success.

Setting SMART Goals

When you are managing any chronic health condition, especially one that touches so many facets of your lifestyle, like prediabetes, it's important to have goals to work toward. Goals not only help you measure progress; they can also be incredibly empowering and motivational when they are set and tracked correctly. However, the wrong kind of goal setting can have the opposite effect. Goals that are unrealistic or too vague, or that don't hold you to any time line for completion may work against you. It may sound counterintuitive, but it may be helpful to initially set your sights low. If you aim for the stars relative to your starting point, you may become easily discouraged if you don't hit that big goal as quickly as you feel you should.

SMART Goals

In the long run, the most effective goals are SMART goals: specific, measurable, action-oriented, realistic, and timely.

Specific

Don't be vague or general. Saying, "I will eat healthier" leaves a lot of room for interpretation. But saying, "I will add one more serving of a low-carb veggie to my meals each day for a week" is a concrete objective you can achieve.

Measurable

Make sure your goals can be measured against something. Whether it's testing blood sugar three more times a week or exercising twenty additional minutes a day, putting a number against your goal helps ensure you're making progress.

Action-Oriented

It may go without saying, but your goal should require you to do something to achieve it. Goals aren't wishes; they are something to work toward by taking tangible steps.

Realistic

Do not set goals you are simply not capable of making or goals that require too much drastic change at once. A realistic goal is something you are fairly certain you can achieve in the short term.

Timely

Set a time limit for your goal. Starting with a short period can be a good motivator for sticking to your goal. As you experience success meeting it, you can always extend the time frame longer.

Goals: What Works and What Doesn't

Not So SMART	What's Missing	The SMART Version
I will test my blood sugar more.	Not measurable or timely	I will test my blood sugar one more time each day for two weeks.
I will start exercising.	Not specific, measurable, or timely	I will walk for twenty minutes at least three days a week for a month.
I will lose 50 pounds this month.	Not action-oriented or realistic	I will lose 3–5 pounds in a month by following the eating and exercise plan I developed with my registered dietitian.
I will take better care of myself.	Not specific, measurable, or timely	By the end of this month, I will make an appointment for my annual dilated eye exam, and I will ask for a reminder call for next year's appointment.
I will have fewer blood sugar swings this month.	Not action-oriented	I will log my sugars, food, meds, and exercise for two weeks and bring it to my doctor to look for patterns that could be causing my blood sugar swings.

Start by picking one goal for yourself. If you're having problems figuring out what the best goal is for you to start with, you can work with your doctor, dietitian, or diabetes educator to narrow down the options.

When You Meet Your Goals

What's the best thing to do once you've met a SMART goal? Get SMARTER, of course! That means evaluating and resetting your goals.

Look at the progress you've made with the original goal. How well did you do in achieving it? Are you satisfied with the results? Are there any changes you could make to do better the next time around in terms of being specific, measurable, action-oriented, realistic, and timely?

If you feel the goal you've worked toward and met has become a healthy new lifestyle habit, then it's time to move on to a new goal (with SMART goal setting in mind, of course). But if your achieved goal isn't quite habit yet, or if the time frame for your goal has elapsed without quite meeting the measurement you set for yourself, you might consider resetting to the same goal—with any modifications you figured out while evaluating your success (e.g., set a different time frame, determine a change in measure).

Remember that you can evaluate and reset goals at any time if you feel like you aren't making adequate progress. Goals should always be a work in progress. And you should always be working toward a goal, even if you've reached your target weight, blood sugars, or other desired health parameters. Doing so will help you stay motivated toward maintaining good health and prevent you from becoming complacent.

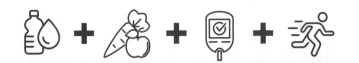

PART II
Develop Habits for Health

Chapter 4

Eat for Your Life

YOU MAY THINK that having prediabetes means you will have to give up everything you like to eat, especially carbohydrates. Nothing could be further from the truth! With the help and advice of a registered dietitian, you can adopt healthy eating habits that fit into your lifestyle. Realize that you won't be able to change your eating habits overnight. It is much easier to adopt the approach of taking small steps every day. Over time, you can make significant changes toward improving your health and reaching near-normal blood glucose levels consistently. To put it simply, a meal plan for managing prediabetes is a plan that most people can follow for good health.

Eat a Balanced Diet

A well-planned and balanced diet that includes a variety of foods can meet all your nutritional needs. Some individuals have other health issues in addition to prediabetes, and this may affect specific nutritional requirements. Discuss all of your health issues with your doctor and registered dietitian to determine whether you should take vitamin and mineral supplements to help meet specific nutritional needs.

All about Carbohydrates

Carbohydrates are your body's primary source of glucose, and glucose is your cellular fuel. The body begins to convert carbohydrates almost entirely into glucose shortly after carb-containing foods are eaten. Insulin helps to "unlock" the cells to move the glucose from the bloodstream into the cells for energy. If you have insufficient insulin production or your body is resistant to insulin, consuming too many carbohydrates can cause blood sugar to rise. Carbohydrates and the glucose they generate are an energy source—the dietary fuel of the human body. Insulin produced by the pancreas enables our cells to burn this carb-generated glucose. This is why determining the amount of carbohydrates in a meal is so important for blood sugar control. Having prediabetes or diabetes does not mean you must cut out all carbohydrates from your diet. You will be happy to learn that there are many carbohydrate food choices that you can include in your plan as long as you maintain an appropriate portion size and choose carbohydrates that have good nutritional value.

All foods that contain starches and/or sugars—including fruits, vegetables, milk, yogurt, breads, grains, beans, and pasta—contain carbs. Simple carbohydrates include sugars, sweets, juices, and fruits. Complex carbohydrates include all types of grain products and starchy vegetables such as potatoes and corn. Virtually the only whole foods that are carbohydrate-free are protein-rich meats, poultry, fish (when prepared without additional ingredients such as breading and marinades), and fats such as cooking oils and butter. To avoid all carb-containing foods is both impossible and unadvisable—your body needs the important micronutrients and plant-based phytochemicals contained in these foods. But you do need to learn the basics of assessing the quantity and quality of carbohydrates in your food, how your body reacts to them, and how to make smart carb choices based on this information.

How Many Carbohydrates Can I Consume?

Despite many studies investigating this topic, the precise amount of carbohydrates to include in the diet for prediabetes and diabetes has not been determined. Your diet will be individualized depending on your weight, activity level, medications, and medical history. The ADA recommends that people with diabetes eat no less than 130 grams of carbs daily. However, many people find that an even lower intake of carbohydrates offers them better control of their blood glucose levels. If you'd like to try a lower-carb meal plan, talk with your RD and your doctor about an approach that's right for you. You can also check Appendix C at the end of this book for helpful online resources for carbohydrate counting information.

For meal planning purposes, carbohydrates are put into five categories. The five groups and example servings are as follows:

1. Starches/Starchy Vegetables: ⅓ cup cooked rice or pasta, 1 slice of bread, ½ cup cooked oatmeal, ½ cup corn or peas, 1 cup butternut squash
2. Fruits: 1 whole piece of fruit (size of tennis ball) like an orange or apple, 1 cup cubed fruit, 17 grapes, 10 cherries
3. Milk/Yogurt: 1 cup milk or 6 ounces light yogurt
4. Non-Starchy Vegetables: 1 cup raw veggies or ½ cup cooked
5. "Other" Carbohydrates: 2 small cookies, ½ cup pudding

The Glycemic Index

Does it matter what kind of carbohydrates you consume? At one time, nutritionists believed that people with diabetes should avoid simple sugars (monosaccharides and disaccharides) and eat foods that contain complex carbohydrates instead. This recommendation was founded on the mistaken belief that simple sugars would raise glucose levels faster and more dramatically across the board. But it's now known that, gram for gram, the complex carbohydrates found in breads, cereals, potatoes, vegetables, and other foods raise blood sugar approximately the same amount as do simple sugars like honey, fructose, or table sugar.

There may be a difference in how rapidly certain foods raise blood sugar levels. The glycemic index (GI) is a measure of how quickly the carbs in certain foods are transformed into blood glucose. Foods with a low GI (e.g., beans, multigrain bread) raise glucose levels at a slower and steadier rate than a high-GI food (e.g., rice, potatoes).

It's important to understand that carbohydrates don't work in isolation. Other nutrient components of the food you eat can also affect your body's ability to absorb carbs. High-fat and high-protein foods can delay carb absorption. And although fiber is considered a carbohydrate, high-fiber foods also slow the absorption of glucose because they slow the passage of food through the digestive tract.

The GI Index

Some complex carbohydrates may have a higher GI than simple carbohydrates. For people with diabetes, the GI can be an effective tool for avoiding blood sugar spikes.

Why Fiber Is Important

Fiber is considered a carbohydrate, but since the body cannot digest the majority of fiber, it does not effectively contribute to a rise in blood sugar levels. There are two types of fiber found in foods: soluble and insoluble. It's important to include foods containing both types of fiber in your daily eating plan.

Soluble Fiber

Soluble fiber dissolves or swells when it's put into water. This type of fiber may help keep blood sugar levels stable by slowing down the rate of glucose absorption into the bloodstream. Soluble fiber absorbs the excess intestinal bile acids that help to form cholesterol, so in turn it helps lower blood cholesterol levels as well. Beans, fruit, barley, and oats are especially good sources of soluble fiber.

Insoluble Fiber

Insoluble fiber does not dissolve in water. In the body, it is not readily broken down by bacteria in the intestinal tract, and this type of fiber passes through the body. Insoluble fiber is essential for preventing constipation and colon health by helping to maintain regularity. Vegetables, whole-grain foods, and fruit are all good sources of insoluble fiber.

The effects of fiber on blood sugar and cholesterol are an important consideration for people with prediabetes/diabetes and who are at risk for cardiovascular disease. In addition, fiber also improves satiety, or the feeling of fullness you get when eating. Soluble fiber delays stomach emptying, and in those people with prediabetes or type 2 diabetes who are also overweight, satiety can be a useful tool for achieving both weight loss and blood sugar control.

When Is a Product Whole Grain?

If a whole-grain ingredient is not listed as the first ingredient, the item may contain only a small portion of whole grains. One way to find a whole-grain product is to look for one of the three "Whole Grain Stamps" from the Whole Grains Council. If a product is labeled "100% Whole Grain," that means that all the grain ingredients are whole grain, with a minimum requirement of 16 grams per serving. The 50%+ stamp indicates that half of the grain ingredients are whole grain, with a minimum of 8 grams per serving. A product with the basic stamp has at least 8 grams of whole grain but may also include some refined grain.

A diet high in low-glycemic whole-grain cereal fiber has been found to have a beneficial effect in controlling postprandial (after-meal) blood glucose levels and for reducing serum cholesterol levels in people with type 2 diabetes. Some studies have shown a glucose- and lipid-lowering benefit with fiber intake of up to 50 grams daily. Fiber intake has also been associated with a reduction in diabetes risk in a number of studies. One of these studies, the six-year Nurses' Health Study, involved more than 65,000 participants and found that women on a low-fiber diet that was heavy in processed sugary foods were 2.5 times more likely to develop type 2 diabetes than those who ate at least 25 grams of fiber daily. The ADA recommends a daily fiber intake of at least 14 grams per 1,000 calories. Talk to your doctor and dietitian about what level of fiber in your diet is right for you.

Drink Water!

The consumption of fiber without adequate fluid intake can lead to constipation. Increasing fiber intake slowly can also help to ease any bloating or other unwanted gastrointestinal distress.

Concerned about Sugar Intake? Get the Facts

The no-sugar myth is probably one of the biggest misconceptions about diabetes. The reality is that it isn't sugar specifically that raises blood glucose levels—it's any food that contains carbohydrates, including honey, fruit, milk, bread, and vegetables, to name a few. Whether it's a spoonful of sugar, a bagel, or a banana, it will cause blood sugar levels to rise. However, some foods may cause a faster or more pronounced blood sugar spike (as previously discussed in the glycemic index section). Sugar isn't, in itself, completely off-limits in a diabetes meal plan. However, moderation in sugar intake is important. Some people with diabetes prefer to use sugar substitutes such as artificial sweeteners or sugar alcohols because they contain few or no carbohydrates or calories.

Sugar Substitutes

Sugar substitutes are never mandatory when you have prediabetes, but they can offer options to those who wish to use them. Using a sugar substitute in a recipe can slash sugar content and a significant number of calories. When using sugar substitutes in baking, keep in mind that sweetness is being added to the food, but other traits unique to a baked product (volume, texture, golden-brown color) may be altered.

Sugar Alcohols

A sugar alcohol is, quite simply, a monosaccharide that has been chemically transformed into its alcohol form. A number of naturally occurring sugar alcohols (also called polyols) are available, including sorbitol, mannitol, xylitol, lactitol, maltitol, isomalt, erythritol, and hydrogenated starch hydrolysates. Because they are not completely absorbed in the gastrointestinal tract, they don't cause much of a rise in blood glucose levels, which is why people with diabetes may find them desirable. Polyols are frequently used as sweeteners and bulking agents in processed foods marketed as sugar-free. It is important not to overdo it with your intake of sugar alcohols because some people find that they have a laxative effect, causing diarrhea and/or gas.

Alternative Sweeteners

The following sweeteners are all approved by the FDA. They vary in taste, uses, and suitability for cooking or baking. You will need to do a taste test on your own to decide which ones are best for you.

SUGAR SUBSTITUTES

Sweetener	Brand Name	Notes
Saccharin	Sweet 'N Low or Sugar Twin	Saccharin can leave a bitter aftertaste and may need to be combined with other sweeteners to improve taste when used in cooking. Twenty-four packets replace 1 cup of sugar.
Aspartame	Equal or NutraSweet	High temperatures diminish sweetness, making this product less suitable for baking. Aspartame contains phenylalanine, which can be harmful to people with the rare disease phenylketonuria (PKU), and it must be avoided by them.
Sucralose	Splenda	There are several baking products using sucralose, including a granular version that measures cup for cup with sugar. There are also half sugar and half brown sugar blends, which contain sugar, so adjust accordingly.
Stevia	Truvia, PureVia	Look for brands of stevia that use a purified portion of the stevia leaf known as rebaudioside A. Sugar to stevia ratios vary with each brand, so follow recommendations by the manufacturer if using in cooking or baking.

Keep in mind that the majority of these sweeteners (with the exception of stevia) are synthetically manufactured and not natural, so it is best to consume them in moderation and not as a complete replacement for whole, natural foods. The sweetener stevia is actually an herb. The Food and Drug Administration (FDA) initially banned the import of stevia in 1991, following a study that raised questions about its toxicity as a food additive. Subsequently, however, the FDA allowed it to be sold as a dietary supplement. In 2008, the FDA allowed food manufacturers to file for generally recognized as safe (GRAS) status for food products made with rebaudioside A (or Reb A). Reb A is a highly purified extract of the stevia herb. There is a body of substantial, controlled research to back up the safety of this extract. The result is that tabletop sweeteners containing this stevia extract can now be sold as food products, not supplements, for the first time. Other foods and beverages sweetened with Reb A can be found on your grocery store shelves. It is important to note that whole-leaf stevia and other stevia extracts are still not FDA-approved for use in food products in the US and can only be found as supplements. If you're considering using a supplement form of stevia, talk with your doctor and dietitian before incorporating it into your food plan.

"Sugar-Free" Is No Guarantee

Don't be misled by a "sugar-free" label. Foods containing polyols and/or artificial sweeteners may still contain carbohydrates and calories that should be figured into your meal plan. Read the nutrition facts on the label to get the full story.

Fats and Cholesterol

Fat insulates the body and supplies energy when no carbohydrate sources are available. It also enables the body to absorb and process the fat-soluble vitamins A, D, E, and K. However, some types of fat and cholesterol may increase the risk of atherosclerosis and other cardiovascular complications from diabetes. Fats are confusing to many people when they first start learning about the dietary management of prediabetes. The off-target message that "all fat is bad" became entrenched in popular dietary culture in the 1990s, turning fat-free food production into a multimillion-dollar industry. While some fats are bad for you in excess, others can actually help improve your cholesterol profile. Here are the basics on dietary fats:

Saturated Fat

This term refers to solid fats found in meat and dairy products and vegetable oils. Too much saturated fat in the diet may be associated with high LDL (bad) cholesterol levels. However, research is conflicting as to whether or not dietary saturated fat actually increases your risk of heart disease, and recent studies dispute this claim.

Unsaturated Fats

These fats are found in plants as well as fish and seafood. These include polyunsaturated fats (e.g., safflower oil, fish, walnuts) or monounsaturated fats (e.g., olive oil, nuts, avocado). These types of fats (polyunsaturated, in particular) have been shown to be effective in reducing total and LDL (bad) cholesterol levels.

Trans Fats/Hydrogenated Fats

This category includes trans unsaturated fatty acids or unsaturated liquid fats that have been processed into a more saturated and solid form by adding hydrogen. These fats are often found in processed baked goods and commercial fried foods and may be called partially hydrogenated or hydrogenated fats. Trans-fatty acids can raise LDL (bad) cholesterol and lower HDL (good) cholesterol, and you should limit your consumption or avoid them altogether.

Omega "Essential" Fatty Acids

These are types of polyunsaturated fat, which have heart-protective benefits and lower both triglyceride levels and blood pressure and are found in fish and fish oils and certain seeds and nuts and their oils (e.g., flaxseed, canola, soybean, and walnut). Linolenic, alpha-linolenic, eicosapentaenoic, and docosahexaenoic acids are all essential fatty acids.

Dietary Cholesterol

Cholesterol is present in food that comes from animals, including poultry, fish, eggs, meats, and dairy products.

How Much Fat Can I Eat?

The National Academy of Medicine has defined an acceptable amount of total fat for all adults to be 20–35 percent of total calorie intake. The type of fat is more important than the total amount consumed when considering cardiovascular risk, so the goal for people with and without diabetes is to have 10 percent or less of daily calories come from saturated fats, and trans fat intake should be limited as much as possible. Cholesterol intake should be less than 200 milligrams per day. The ADA also recommends two or more servings of fish weekly for the cardioprotective benefits of omega-3 fatty acids. Examples of fat servings would be: 1 teaspoon of butter or margarine, ⅛ of a medium avocado, or 1 tablespoon of salad dressing or oil.

Protein: Your Building Blocks to Good Health

Proteins are chains of amino acids responsible for cell growth and maintenance and are found in virtually every part of the body. Protein in foods from animal sources (meat, poultry, fish, and dairy) is called complete protein because it contains essential amino acids necessary for building and maintaining cells. Protein in plant-based foods such as grains, beans, fruit, and vegetables is called incomplete protein because it contains only partial groups of these amino acids. However, different incomplete plant-based proteins can be combined to form complete proteins in your diet. If you are a vegetarian or vegan and have prediabetes, a dietitian with experience in vegetarian menu planning can advise you on appropriate protein consumption choices.

How Much Protein Should You Eat?

Protein intake goals should also be individualized, but a ballpark suggestion is that people with prediabetes should have 15–20 percent of total calories from protein, as is recommended for the general population. Some research has suggested that higher protein diets with 20–30 percent of calories from protein may be beneficial to help with feeling full longer.

People with impaired kidney function, or nephropathy, may need to avoid a high-protein diet because damaged kidneys cannot filter protein efficiently from the bloodstream. If you have kidney problems, talk to your doctor and dietitian about an appropriate level of protein for your diet. Examples of protein servings would be: 3–5 ounces of chicken, fish, pork, or red meat; ½ cup tofu; 1 egg; or ¼ cup cottage cheese.

Sensible Sodium Intake

In moderate amounts, dietary sodium or sodium chloride (salt) is not harmful. In fact, this mineral helps to maintain a healthy electrolyte balance and works in tandem with potassium to regulate blood acid/base balance, heart function, nerve impulses, and muscle contractions. However, people with high blood pressure need to be cautious about having too much sodium in their daily diet. The Dietary Approaches to Stop Hypertension (or DASH diet) study found that limiting dietary sodium is associated with a substantial reduction in blood pressure in adults with hypertension.

How Much Sodium Am I Allowed?

For most people with diabetes and hypertension, the ADA recommends a daily sodium intake of 2,300 milligrams, equivalent to a teaspoon of sodium chloride, or table salt. The average American, however, consumes more than twice that much. Watch out for added sodium in condiments and packaged and canned foods. Some people with hypertension may benefit from an even bigger cut in dietary salt intake. Studies have shown that reducing sodium intake to 1,500 milligrams or less daily reduces blood pressure significantly when it is part of a comprehensive DASH diet—a dietary approach that is low in saturated fat and cholesterol and rich in fiber, protein, calcium, magnesium, and potassium.

What about Alcohol?

When it comes to alcohol and your health, the optimal word is always moderation. Consider the facts about alcohol and decide whether including alcohol on a moderate basis fits into your prediabetes management plan. Alcohol does not provide any essential nutrients, but it is a source of calories. If you drink and are having difficulty losing weight, do not overlook the calories that alcohol adds to your overall intake. Alcohol can impact blood lipid levels and elevate triglycerides. Both of these health issues may already be a source of concern for you.

It is perfectly okay to add a small amount of alcohol in certain recipes. A bit of wine or flavored liqueur can enhance the flavor of the food and can be incorporated as a low-fat cooking ingredient or marinade. When cooked, the alcohol content diminishes, but the flavor remains.

Putting It All Together: Meal Planning

A meeting with a registered dietitian (RD) is an absolute must for anyone with prediabetes. A good RD will explain the different food categories (carbohydrates, protein, fats) to you in more detail and will work with you to create a meal plan that works with your lifestyle. If you don't have an RD already, talk to your doctor about a referral, or visit the Academy of Nutrition and Dietetics's online referral database at www.eatright.org.

Vitamin and Mineral Supplements

Eating a balanced diet that includes foods from all the essential food groups generally meets the nutrition needs of most adults. Some individuals have other health issues in addition to prediabetes, and this may affect specific nutritional requirements. Discuss all your health issues with your doctor and registered dietitian to determine whether you should take vitamin and mineral supplements to help meet specific nutritional needs.

In addition, one easy way to plan meals is using the plate method. The plate method, a.k.a. MyPlate, is the most current food guide developed by the US Department of Agriculture (USDA), which replaced the Food

Guide Pyramid in 2011. With the plate method, you fill half of your plate with non-starchy vegetables, a quarter of your plate with protein, and the remaining quarter of your plate with grains and starchy foods. You can add a serving of fruit, dairy, or both, as your meal plan allows, as well as a low-calorie beverage. For more information about the plate method, visit: www.choosemyplate.gov. See Appendix C for more online resources with information on meal planning, the plate method, and carbohydrate counting.

Now that you have a basic background on nutrition and prediabetes, it is time to put it into practice. The following are some important habits to adopt that provide specific suggestions and action steps you can take to make positive changes in your eating to promote blood sugar control and overall good health.

1. Be Savvy with Your Starches

Starches provide the body with energy, but you want to be sure not to overdo it on portions or starchy foods that can translate to high blood sugars later. Keep starch portions to a quarter of your plate and choose whole-grain varieties that are high in fiber. The best way to get more whole grains in your meals is to substitute refined products with whole-grain foods. Gradually start replacing the refined grains in your kitchen cabinets with whole-grain foods and consume moderate portions.

Tips to Make the Habit Stick

- When a recipe calls for white flour (all-purpose), experiment by replacing some of the flour with a whole-grain variety.
- Use a whole grain as a side dish or mix it with vegetables, lentils, or beans.
- Every week try one "new" grain that you have not used before. Quinoa, brown rice, bulgur, or kasha may be unfamiliar to you, but these grains are as easy to prepare as white rice.
- Add whole grains like brown rice, barley, or quinoa to soups, salads, or casseroles instead of white rice or pasta.
- Choose a cooked whole grain as a hot breakfast cereal, like oats or multigrain blends, or try a baked oatmeal recipe.
- If you are not used to bran or other high-fiber cereals, try mixing them with equal amounts of your regular cereal.
- Switch to whole-grain crackers instead of saltines or other white-flour snack crackers.
- Use rolled oats or whole-wheat bread crumbs in items such as meatloaf or meatballs.

2. Fill Up on Non-Starchy Veggies

Pile half your plate with raw and/or cooked veggies to achieve satiety and keep your nutrient and fiber intake high and your calories and carb counts low in order to promote blood sugar and weight control. There are a lot of great ways to increase the portions of vegetables in your family meals. Be creative to get in plenty of veggies daily.

Tips to Make the Habit Stick

- Toss shredded carrots with spaghetti or stir canned pumpkin into pasta sauce. Or bake a veggie lasagna. You can even blend veggies into your marinara or pizza sauce.
- Blanket veggies like zucchini, broccoli, and mushrooms into quesadillas or scramble them into an omelet.
- Construct a festive burrito or tostada bowl with black beans, brown rice, cheese, avocado, and tomato salsa.
- Bake shredded zucchini and carrot into quick breads and muffins.
- Simmer generous portions of carrots and celery in chicken noodle or rice soup, or try puréed soups such as carrot or butternut squash. Make a stew with meat and veggies.
- Top thin-crust pizza with plenty of veggies like mushrooms and peppers.
- Blend veggies like carrots (even spinach!) into a fruit smoothie.
- Use cauliflower steamed and mashed/puréed as faux mashed potatoes or chopped very fine and cooked as a rice substitute.
- Add chopped veggies like carrots, peppers, and mushrooms into your meatloaf, burgers, or meatballs (use lean ground turkey to start with to trim the saturated fat).

3. Do Your Dairy Wisely and in Moderation

Both the ADA and the USDA recommend consuming low-fat rather than full-fat dairy products. Traditionally this recommendation has been based on the presumed link between saturated fat and heart disease, but more research is being conducted regularly to see if we really need to shy away entirely from saturated fat. For now, get in the habit of limiting full-fat dairy to small amounts and know that low-fat dairy products such as cheese, cottage cheese, yogurt, and milk are lower in fat and calories. They help with satiety, and they are good sources of calcium for bone health, as well as protein for muscle mass. Be aware that a cup of milk or light yogurt has 12 grams of carbs. You need to account for that in your carb budget so you can keep your blood sugars in check. If you cannot digest or are allergic to dairy, you can choose soy or almond milk/yogurt alternatives, but make it a priority to check the ingredient lists for added sugar and too many other additives.

Tips to Make the Habit Stick

- Keep cheese portions to an ounce—a slice of cheese on a sandwich or a ¼ cup of shredded cheese on a salad can go a long way.

- Regular yogurt, namely fruit-flavored, can have a ton of carbs and sugar, so keep to the "light" varieties or, better yet, buy plain, unsweetened yogurt and add your own fresh fruit to prevent an unwanted spike in blood sugars later.

- Newly popular Greek yogurt, which is strained to be higher in protein and lower in carbs, is also a great choice.

4. Feast on Fruits in Their Natural Form

When it comes to fruit, whole and fresh is the best choice. That way you get all the nutrients and fiber without added sugar. Fruits contain natural sugars (fructose) that raise blood sugar levels, yet they also have fiber to help moderate that effect. It's all about choosing fresh fruit and watching portions. Fruits especially high in fiber include: watermelon, strawberries, grapefruit, blackberries, blueberries, and honeydew melon. No fruits are off-limits as long as you watch your portions. Savor a variety of fresh fruit—spread it out daily and eat it in sensible portions.

Tips to Make the Habit Stick

- Enjoy 2–3 servings of fruit per day but spread them out during the day at meals and snacks.
- Have a piece of fruit as a snack, top plain yogurt, cereal, or salads with fresh berries, or try a tasty seasonal fruit salad as a refreshing dessert.
- Remember to minimize fruit juices, canned fruits in syrup and juices, and all dried fruits (e.g., raisins, prunes, dates, dried apricots) because they are extremely high in sugar.

5. Pump Up the Protein...Lean, That Is

The good news is, when prepared without sauces or breading, meat, poultry, and fish are all carbohydrate-free and chock-full of protein that will help keep you full for weight control and won't spike your blood sugars. Aim to include a good source of protein at each meal.

Tips to Make the Habit Stick

- Go for lean options such as chicken and turkey breast without skin, pork loin/chops, and white fish. Choosing lean cuts of red meat like sirloin tip or top round (cuts that have less fat marbled within the meat) will also help you avoid some of the added fat and calories. Also, cooking meat dishes in low-fat ways such as baking, steaming, or grilling helps keep them healthy choices.

- As with all food, fresh and natural is best. Minimize cured, smoked, and processed meats (such as bacon, sausage, and deli meats), which are full of sodium and additives like nitrates.

- There are few exceptions to lean protein that are still healthy, such as nuts/nut butter and fatty fish (like tuna and salmon), which contain healthy fats. Nut butters work great for sandwiches or spread on whole-grain crackers, celery, and apple slices.

- Beans and legumes are a cheap, easy source of plant protein and are also full of soluble fiber. A ½-cup serving of beans contains about 15 grams of carbohydrates in addition to its 7 grams of protein. Use beans in soups, atop salads, or as a high-fiber starch side dish.

- Tofu can be a good vegetarian source of protein, but watch out for soy-based commercial meat substitutes because many are processed with sodium and other additives.

6. Embrace Healthy Fats in Small Doses

More and more research has shown that the "fat-free" trend of the nineties is no longer the way to go and including healthy plant-based fats in small portions can help with satiety and add flavor and healthy nutrients as well as provide some protective benefits as far as prediabetes, diabetes, and heart disease are concerned. Try to have a dab of healthy fat at each meal, but don't overdo it. Fats will not increase blood sugar, but they are high in calories, so keep your portions small to avoid unwanted weight gain. Fats contain over twice as many calories per gram as protein and carbs, so overdoing it on portions can add to your waistline.

Tips to Make the Habit Stick

- Two great healthy fat options include nuts and avocado. Add 1–2 tablespoons of avocado to your salad, in omelets, or spread on toast. Enjoy a small handful of nuts as a snack or sprinkle them (or sunflower seeds) on your morning cereal or atop salads.
- Keep your oil use in check. Even though plant-based oils like olive and canola contain heart-healthy unsaturated fat, using too much in cooking can easily add a lot of calories to seemingly low-calorie food such as veggies.

7. Shy Away from Salt

Remember that the current *Dietary Guidelines for Americans* recommends a sodium intake for healthy adults of no more than 2,300 milligrams of sodium per day. Achieving this goal is particularly challenging for individuals who rely on packaged or processed foods as a large part of their diet. By reducing consumption of processed foods and including more whole, natural, and fresh foods, you can reduce your daily sodium consumption. While salt will not increase blood pressure in many people, it can increase blood pressure in some people, so moderate intake is recommended. There are still plenty of ways you can spice things up and flavor your food that don't involve salt.

Tips to Make the Habit Stick

- Leave out or reduce the amount of salt in standard recipes by 25–50 percent.
- Use low-sodium condiments and flavorings like fresh basil, lemon, pepper, garlic, mustard, salsa, vinegars, and commercial herb blends to season food instead of using salt.
- Limit intake of highly processed foods such as boxed mixes, instant foods, snack foods, and processed meats.
- Make more soups, stews, casseroles, or side dishes from scratch.
- Watch your use of the saltshaker when cooking or at the table.

8. Think about What You Drink

You may already know that it's important to drink plenty of fluids throughout the day, but you also need to pay attention to the quality of your fluids, not just the quantity. Water is your best bet because it hydrates you simply, without anything added. Focus on consuming water as your main source of hydration to cut calories, sugar, and additives. Try to keep what you drink as simple as possible.

Tips to Make the Habit Stick

- Avoid sodas, fruit juices, smoothies, and/or sweetened coffee drinks; these are sources of empty calories and sugar that can wreak havoc on your blood glucose levels and waistline. Instead, go for decaffeinated black tea or coffee and sparkling water with a squeeze of lemon.
- Drink alcohol in moderation, limiting it to special occasions if you can, to cut excess empty calories. If you do have a drink, good choices are light beer, a skinny margarita, a Bloody Mary, a rum and Coke (with diet cola), a 5-ounce glass of red wine, or a vodka with seltzer instead of tonic water.
- Limit drinks with artificial sweeteners (or avoid them entirely if you can) to minimize consuming chemicals.

9. Practice Portion Control

It's a good idea to measure most foods and beverages you consume until you get a feel for portion sizes. That way you are less likely to overdo it, which can lead to higher blood sugars and excess weight. It's a supersized world out there, and most people are surprised to find that their idea of a single serving is actually two or three. The only tools you really need are a simple and inexpensive gram scale, dry and liquid measuring cups, and measuring spoons. Try to measure and guesstimate your portions regularly.

Tips to Make the Habit Stick

- Early on, it's a good idea to run everything that isn't premeasured through a scale, cup, or spoon first. That way you will get really good at eyeballing portions when you eat out.
- There are also plenty of nifty tricks for estimating portion sizes, such as:
  - A cup of fruit or yogurt = a baseball, a clenched fist, or a small apple
  - 3 ounces of fish, meat, or poultry = a deck of cards, the palm of your hand, or a pocket pack of tissues
  - 1 teaspoon of butter or mayonnaise = a thimble or the head of a toothbrush
  - 1 tablespoon of peanut butter = the size of your thumb
  - 1 ounce of cheese = a tube of lip balm an AA battery, or a domino

10. Be Healthy on a Budget

Eating right doesn't have to be expensive. You don't have to spend tons of money to stick to a sensible meal plan for your prediabetes. Don't be afraid to clip coupons. There are many ways to choose a variety of healthy foods that still fit your budget.

Tips to Make the Habit Stick

- Buy whole grains and other staples in bulk. Avoid snack packs and single portions; you can buy in bulk and preportion at home.

- Many places offer generic brands or their own store-brand versions of popular whole-grain cereals and breads, so stock up on these to keep costs down.

- Making your own homemade baked goods is cheaper and healthier too, since you can use whole-grain flour and cut down on the sugar. Shop for fruits and veggies in season, as these will likely be on sale and taste the best.

- Buying whole-leaf greens and rinsing them yourself in a salad spinner can often cut costs over bagged salads.

- Try some great canned fruits and veggie choices such as pumpkin, beets, tomatoes, and pineapple packed in juice (rinsed).

- Buying fresh frozen fruits and veggies is a great way to get them year-round at low cost, and they don't have any added sodium or sugar. Buy milk, yogurt, cheese, cottage cheese, eggs, and fresh meats on sale weekly to keep costs down.

- Dried or canned beans are cheap and full of protein and fiber. A large jar of peanut butter will last awhile for sandwiches and snacks.

11. Shop Smart

Being prepared and in the right frame of mind can make all the difference when you are shopping for food. Never go to the grocery store hungry because this can set you up to give in to the temptation to buy less-healthy food. Take the time to plan ahead before you grocery shop to stay on track.

Tips to Make the Habit Stick

- Go shopping after a meal or have a small, wholesome snack like a piece of fruit or string cheese before you head out.
- Make a list of foods that fit your prediabetes meal plan so you can arrive prepared and maximize your time while in the store. Create a basic list on the computer to print or have one ready on your smartphone that you can keep and add to throughout the year so you do not have to "re-create the wheel" each time you hit the store aisles.

12. Go Ahead, Dine Out! But Within Your Meal Plan

Keep it clean and simple when eating out. Planning ahead, making smart substitutions and good menu choices can help you keep within the scope of your meal plan.

Tips to Make the Habit Stick

- Remember to use the plate method (plate = ¼ protein, ¼ starch, and ½ non-starchy veggies) when making food choices.
- Skip the bread basket or chips and start with a salad or broth-based soup instead.
- Request that all condiments be served on the side.
- If you have a taste for the steak dinner, swap the potato for a double serving of salad or veggies instead.
- Avoid breaded items and anything fried or sautéed in heavy oil/butter. The best restaurant menu picks include:
  - Dishes prepared with tomato sauces rather than cream sauces
  - Grilled, poached, or broiled fish or poultry dishes
  - Grilled or broiled meats served without gravies or sauces
  - Vegetables that have been steamed or lightly sautéed or grilled
  - High-fiber starches such as brown rice, whole-wheat pasta, baked potato with the skin (but keep portions to ¼ plate)
  - Broth-based soups instead of cream soups
  - Salads with dressing on the side and minus the extras such as cheese and croutons
- And for dessert? Order a single item for the table and just have a bite or two, order fruit, or enjoy a sugar-free hard candy or a small healthy dessert within your meal plan waiting for you at home. See Appendix B at the end of this book for more healthy dining out details.

13. Snack Sensibly

Snacks are a great way to keep you energized and to prevent excess hunger as well as overeating at mealtimes, but don't get sabotaged by a snack attack gone haywire. Too much snacking, particularly eating the wrong foods, can send your blood sugars and weight out of control. Choosing the right snacks to have between meals can make all the difference in helping you along with your meal plan.

Tips to Make the Habit Stick

- Plan ahead to keep healthy snacks readily available in your cupboard or on the go. That way you won't just grab or buy whatever is in sight when hunger hits.

- It can be helpful to consume snacks that are high in fiber, as well as mini combos of protein and fat to help satisfy you and keep your blood sugar more stable until the next mealtime. Good high-fiber choices include a piece of whole fruit, ¾ cup berries, ¼ cup shelled edamame (soybeans), 3 cups air-popped popcorn, or raw veggies with low-fat ranch dressing.

- If you are looking for a heartier snack with carb plus protein, try ½ apple spread with 1 tablespoon peanut butter, 6 ounces of Greek yogurt with ¼ cup fresh fruit, 5 whole-grain crackers with an ounce of cheese, or a rice cake spread with 2 tablespoons of hummus.

- Want a low-carb alternative? A stick of low-fat string cheese or a handful of nuts or celery sticks with peanut butter will do.

14. Investigate Ingredients Lists—Less Is More

Keep it simple and natural as far as your prediabetes meal plan is concerned. Steer clear of processed foods as often as you can; a long list of ingredients should be a red flag. Cut down on packaged foods that may have additives such as sugar and salt, not to mention tons of stabilizers and chemicals that you may not even be able to pronounce.

Tips to Make the Habit Stick

- You can take the guesswork out of food choices by choosing whole and natural foods like fresh fruits and veggies; whole-grain staples like oatmeal, brown rice, and corn tortillas; and fresh meats and poultry; as well as nuts and natural nut butters, to name a few examples.

- Try to eat more fresh food that you can prepare yourself at home.

15. Learn the Food Label Lingo

Looking at nutrition fact labels can be overwhelming and confusing at times. Luckily the FDA is continually trying to improve the nutrition facts label. It was last revised in 2016 to reflect updated information about nutrition and science and to make it a bit easier to read. Take time to read and understand labels so you get to know your food better.

Tips to Make the Habit Stick

- Focus on key components on the label such as serving size, amount of nutrients per serving, and the ingredient list:

  - Serving size: Each label must identify the size of a serving. The nutritional information listed on a label is based on one serving of the food.
  - Amount per serving: Each package identifies the quantities of nutrients and food constituents from one serving.
  - Percent daily value: This indicates how much of a specific nutrient a serving of food contains in comparison to an average 2,000-calorie diet.
  - Ingredient list: This is a listing of the ingredients in a food in descending order of predominance and weight.

- You may see that there are several parts to the carbohydrate section of the nutrition label. Total carbohydrate represents the amount of carbohydrate grams found in a food. Beneath the total carbohydrate line are other listings: fiber, sugars, added sugars, and, sometimes, sugar alcohols. Realize that these values are all part of total carbohydrate.

16. Cook Creatively to Keep Healthy

There are many ways to prepare foods that not only preserve nutrients and good taste but also minimize the use of sugar, salt, and fat. A little creativity with spices, herbs, or combining foods together in unconventional ways makes food more flavorful without the addition of extra fat, sodium, or calories. Try new ways to cook healthy at home. Preparing your foods in healthy ways can ensure that your home-cooked meals are in accordance with your meal plan for prediabetes.

Tips to Make the Habit Stick

- Stir-frying, broiling, and slow cooking are examples of techniques that are time-saving and result in more healthful food. Stir-frying uses a very small amount of oil and cooks foods quickly at a high heat. It allows you to combine several foods together for a quick and healthy meal. Foods that work well using the stir-fry method include vegetables, poultry, meats, fish, and cooked grains. Broiling or grilling involves cooking foods on a rack to allow fats to drip to a pan or flame below. Most meats, poultry, or fish can be grilled or broiled. Broiling instead of cooking in oil can reduce fat and calories.

- Slow cookers are now very popular again and with reason. They are extremely easy to use and can save a lot of time in the kitchen when trying to cook healthy. You place foods in the slow cooker early in the day and allow them to cook at a low temperature for several hours or more. Meals made in a slow cooker do not require the addition of fats, and the slow cooking helps tenderize tougher cuts of meat. Soups, sauces, and stews are just a few examples of the items you can cook in a slow cooker.

17. Bake to Help Lower Sugar and Fat

Baking at home helps you control the sugar, fat, and calories to help your favorite recipes coincide with healthy eating for prediabetes control. There are a variety of ways to modify recipes to stick with your meal plan but still enjoy plenty of flavor.

Tips to Make the Habit Stick

- Try reducing a standard recipe's sugar content by 25–50 percent. It's usually best to start with a smaller reduction (25 percent) and gradually decrease the amount of sugar each time the product is made. Be sure to note whether the properties of the food have any significant or undesirable changes, then adjust as needed.

- Use puréed, unsweetened fruit or fruit juices to replace some or all of the sugar in a recipe. Honey or maple syrup are sugars and will affect blood sugar; however, either can add sweetness to a food. Carbohydrates and calories can be reduced if you use a smaller amount of these sugars in a recipe.

- Many recipes can withstand up to a 50 percent reduction in fat. To replace fat, but not volume, try using plain yogurt, applesauce, mashed ripe banana, or other puréed fruit for half of the oil or shortening called for in a recipe. If the product requires sweetness in addition to volume, applesauce or mashed ripe banana make good options.

18. Use Your Recipe Resources

Stumped when trying to think of more ideas to add variety and flavor to your meal plan? Find new healthy recipes by using your resources. You would be surprised at how many healthy recipes are out there. If you search for them, you will find them, in a book, a magazine, or online.

Tips to Make the Habit Stick

- Take advantage of all the recipe information that is out there on the Internet and at your local library.
- Make a goal to try a new recipe every week to mix things up and keep your prediabetes meal plan exciting.
- Swap healthy recipes with family and friends who are in your support network.
- Take a healthy cooking class or subscribe to a magazine that features healthy recipes to motivate you to try new ideas.

19. Venture Into the World of Vinegars and Fermented Foods

The acetic acid in vinegar moderates blood sugar response and also contributes to a feeling of fullness following a meal, which may in turn cause you to eat less. This also holds true for fermented foods such as olives, sauerkraut, kimchi, and pickles (which are not technically fermented but are pickled in vinegar brine).

Tips to Make the Habit Stick

- Most vinegars are blood-sugar friendly, so try them out to add flavor. Dressing salads or veggies with oil and vinegar is an easy way to work vinegar into your dietary repertoire. To increase the effect, add a little lemon juice to the mix, which also helps moderate blood sugar with its high acidity.
- You can marinate proteins such as fish, beef, and chicken in a vinegar mixture. There are many flavors and varieties of vinegar to choose from; if you choose a vinaigrette or a fruit-based vinegar, be sure to check the total carbohydrates on the label to make sure you aren't canceling out the benefits of this versatile and normally low-calorie and low-carbohydrate condiment.
- Use olives, sauerkraut, kimchi, and pickles as side condiments to complement your meals while getting the benefits of dietary acetic acid. Be aware that some of them are considerable sources of sodium, so keeping the portions small is important.

20. Consider Cinnamon

Cinnamon certainly has some potential to be beneficial for those with prediabetes/diabetes. Studies have shown conflicting results as to whether or not cinnamon can help lower your blood sugar levels. Most animal studies have shown a benefit, while human studies have been less conclusive. However, a 2012 meta-analysis published in *The American Journal of Clinical Nutrition* found that cinnamon had beneficial effects on both fasting blood sugar levels and HbA1c, at least up to four months of use. Cinnamon intake for this study ranged between 1 and 6 grams daily, which is a lot of cinnamon. More research on this spice is needed to develop better guidelines on how helpful cinnamon is. But trying a little cinnamon here and there in your diet can't hurt, and it might even help.

Tips to Make the Habit Stick

- Add an extra sprinkle of cinnamon in your coffee, yogurt, fruit, and other cinnamon-friendly foods.
- Steer clear of any cinnamon supplements until more conclusive research about safety and efficacy has been established.

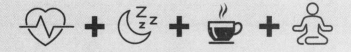

Chapter 5

Move It! Exercise for Your Life

BEING MORE ACTIVE is an important part of your prediabetes plan. One of the simplest and most effective ways to bring down blood sugar levels, cut the risk of cardiovascular disease, and improve overall health and well-being is exercise. Despite these benefits, exercise is a tough sell in our increasingly sedentary world where almost every essential task can be performed online, from the driver's seat, or with a phone call. Redefining your preconceived notions of exercise, and making it fun, is the best way to ensure that you look forward to exercising instead of finding ways to avoid it.

The Importance of Exercise

Everyone should exercise, yet the National Health Interview Survey tells us that less than half of the US adult population gets the recommended thirty minutes of daily physical activity—and 33 percent aren't active at all. Inactivity is thought to be one of the key reasons for the surge of prediabetes and type 2 diabetes in the US—because inactivity and obesity promote insulin resistance.

The good news is that it's never too late to get moving, and exercise is one of the easiest ways to start controlling your prediabetes. Exercise is beneficial to health in a multitude of ways. It promotes blood sugar control to manage prediabetes and can improve other aspects of your health as well.

How Does Exercise Help Control Blood Sugar?

Regular activity and exercise will improve your blood glucose levels. Lower blood glucose levels are achieved when the glucose in your blood is used for energy during and after exercise. Muscle cells become more sensitive to insulin, allowing for better storage and usage of glucose for energy. Cells in the liver also become more sensitive to insulin, and this helps prevent the liver from producing too much glucose. In essence, insulin resistance improves with regular exercise, and gradually blood glucose levels go down. Routine exercise is vital to the process of stopping prediabetes from progressing to diabetes and also for improving your general health.

What Are Some Additional Health Benefits of Exercise?

Exercise does much more than just improve insulin sensitivity and promote blood sugar control. Regular activity also aids in weight loss, maintains bone health, lowers stress, increases balance and flexibility, and helps with sleep. Overall benefits of physical activity, as shown in countless studies, include reduced rates of mortality, cardiovascular disease, hypertension, stroke, certain cancers, Alzheimer's disease, and type 2 diabetes. As far as your health is concerned, there are quite a few reasons to work regular exercise into your day.

How Do You Get Started?

When you first learned you might have prediabetes, your doctor probably encouraged you to begin exercising. If this was not initially discussed, you should talk to your doctor to make sure that exercise is appropriate for you. In most cases, your doctor will support your desire to start an exercise plan. If you have other health issues in addition to prediabetes, you and your doctor should discuss the best types of exercise for you. Be realistic when choosing exercises for yourself. Once your doctor has given you the okay to start, it's time to consider the variables that will help you choose the right type of exercise:

- Consider your physical ability to perform certain activities and choose ones that you can do. Some exercises may be too difficult or strenuous for your current level of fitness.
- Include activities you enjoy or increase those already performed on a semi-regular basis. Going for a walk, gardening, or vacuuming are all activities that can easily help get you moving and be part of your daily routine.
- Think about how much time you have. An ambitious exercise plan that involves too much time will quickly be abandoned if you lack the time.
- If you have not exercised recently, ease into a program that includes short periods to start with.

- Consider the resources available to you. If you do not have access to a gym, exercise equipment, or a pool, then a simple walking plan may be your best bet.

Do You Need to Buy a Lot of Exercise Equipment?

Resist the temptation to purchase home exercise equipment until you have tried it out and are reasonably sure that you will use it. Many types of home equipment end up at garage sales or just taking up space because the owner stopped using the equipment after a short time. If you are considering buying home exercise equipment, try it out first in the store, at a gym, or at a friend's house before purchasing it. Make sure you like the activity enough that you will want to do it often!

When you make plans for exercise and activity, it is important to be honest about your likelihood to maintain the plan. Make sure to plan activities that you will enjoy or do not mind doing. Would you prefer to exercise alone or with the company of a friend or spouse? Will your activity involve being outdoors or indoors? Can you perform the activity outdoors year-round or will you need to find an alternate indoor activity for part of the year? Try to work out any barriers ahead of time that could get in the way of your exercise plan.

How Much Should You Exercise?

In 2011, the American Diabetes Association and the American College of Sports Medicine released joint exercise guidelines for people with type 2 diabetes. The guidelines recommend a minimum of 150 minutes of moderate-intensity aerobic exercise weekly, spread out over at least three days each week. Ideally, no more than two days should pass between aerobic exercise sessions. With younger and more physically fit individuals, shorter durations (minimum seventy-five minutes per week) of vigorous-intensity or interval training may be enough. In addition to aerobic activity, resistance training is also recommended two to three times a week, except for individuals who have other health conditions or complications that make resistance exercise unadvisable.

Exercise Intensity

How hard you should push yourself during exercise depends on your level of fitness and your health history. Your doctor can recommend an optimal heart rate target for working out based on those factors. It's very important to get this information from your doctor before starting an exercise program, especially if you have a history of cardiovascular problems. On average, most people should aim for a target heart rate zone of 50 to 75 percent of their maximum heart rate. Maximum heart rate is computed by subtracting your age from the number 220. So, if you are 40, your maximum heart rate would be 180, and your target heart rate zone would be between 90 and 135 beats per minute.

You should wear a digital or analog watch with a second hand or function to check your heart rate during exercise. To calculate your heart rate, place your fingers at your wrist or neck pulse point and count the number of beats for fifteen seconds. Multiply that number by four to get your heart rate. The number you get should be within your target zone. If it's too high, take your intensity down a few notches. If you're exercising below your target zone, pick things up. If you are new to exercise, you should aim for the lower (50 percent) range of your target heart rate. As you become more fit, you can work toward the 75 percent maximum.

Resistance Training

In addition to aerobic exercise, it is important to incorporate resistance training into your routine, if possible. Resistance training is strength training that works the muscles. Activities such as weight lifting, working with resistance bands, water workouts, and body weight resistance exercises (e.g., push-ups, pull-ups, squats) are all good forms of resistance training. Studies have shown that increasing muscle mass through strength training reduces insulin resistance and helps to lower blood glucose. Resistance exercises should work all the major muscle groups of the upper body, lower body, and core. If you include strength training, be sure to allow at least forty-eight hours between sessions so your muscles are able to rest and recover. For most people, short strength-training sessions two to three times weekly will provide added benefit. If you are new to resistance training, it can be helpful to work with a certified trainer for at least a few sessions to determine the right set of exercises for you and to ensure proper form to get the maximum benefits without risking injury.

Stretching

Stretching is another worthwhile addition to a well-rounded exercise plan because it helps to increase flexibility and prevent injury. Stretch slowly, without bouncing, and only stretch as far as you can without causing any pain. A few minutes of stretching at the beginning and end of an exercise session can make exercise easier and reduce the possibility of injury. Stretching has not been shown to have much impact on glucose control, so it should not be substituted for aerobic or resistance activity but rather used as an add-on to your workout as a whole.

Making Time for Exercise

Your exercise routine should be planned to fit naturally into your daily schedule. Look at your daily routine, then decide where you can realistically fit in some time for activity. If you have a busy schedule, short periods of time (ten to thirty minutes) will probably work much better than trying to carve out an hour for daily activity. Start out with small amounts of time one or more times a day. You will likely have more success getting in activity this way. The habits section of this chapter has plenty of helpful tips for you to incorporate activity into your day.

The Best Time of Day to Exercise

As long as you exercise, the time of day you actually do the exercise is the best time! Busy and demanding schedules often get in the way of good intentions. If your schedule is particularly demanding, try making an appointment on your schedule for your exercise time. Remember that any time spent exercising is better than no time.

No Exercise = Little to No Results

If you really want to stop prediabetes in its tracks, it is important to understand just how important it is to initiate a plan for physical activity. Many people just focus on changing their eating habits. While this is very important, the lack of exercise could prevent you from reaching your goals. Cutting down on food will not be enough to help you lose weight and maintain a lower weight. Physical activity is a key component to your prediabetes plan and must be included at whatever level you are able to accommodate. Exercise is often left out of a health plan because of perceived barriers that keep people from becoming more active. If you are someone who never seems able to find the time or energy for exercise, begin to take a serious look at what the barriers are. Once you identify what is getting in your way, plan strategies to help you go around those barriers. Keep your strategies simple and real. Writing down and implementing your strategy is a good way to help you make permanent changes.

Pregnancy, Children, Disabled, and Obese

Virtually anyone who has the capability to move can exercise to some degree. Activity plans can be developed for individuals in a variety of specific situations and life stages such as pregnancy, in youth, the elderly, or those with particular health conditions. If you are in one of these populations, a doctor can recommend a level and form of exercise that is appropriate for you.

Exercise During Pregnancy

Regular exercise by those who are pregnant with GDM or prediabetes can help promote the physical well-being of the mother and baby. A physician-approved exercise plan can help with blood sugar control and excess weight gain and can provide many other health benefits such as improved cardiovascular fitness and normal blood pressure. In addition, physical activity helps to prevent excess weight in the developing baby, may help prevent preterm birth, and can lead to a healthier weight in the child later in life. Safety is the utmost concern when beginning an exercise routine while pregnant, so it is important to consult with your doctor if you are pregnant to get the go-ahead to begin exercising and to develop an individualized plan that will be right for you.

How to Help Your Children Become More Active

For children and teens, physical activity is an essential part of a healthy lifestyle, helps promote blood sugar control, and may prevent many chronic diseases. Unfortunately, today's children and teens are much less physically active than their parents were. Bicycle riding and jumping rope have been replaced with computer games and phone texting. To get your child's cooperation, help him understand why exercise has to become a regular part of his life. Be positive and emphasize the benefits such as:

- Exercise is essential for keeping a body healthy and strong and for building lean muscle.
- Individuals who are active and fit sustain far fewer illnesses or injuries.
- Physical activity is necessary for maintenance of normal weight.
- Exercise can help with better sleep and is effective for reducing stress.
- Perhaps the most important reason for a child with prediabetes to get exercise: it helps to bring blood glucose back to normal.

Suggested Physical Activity Levels for Kids

Children and teens need about sixty minutes of exercise at least five days a week. If this seems like a lot of time, consider the amount of time they may be spending watching TV or using the computer, video games, or cell phones. For most children, those activities add up to almost seven and a half hours a day!

It is perfectly okay to break sixty minutes of physical activity into shorter intervals during the day. For example, thirty minutes of gym class at school could be complemented with thirty minutes of play outside after school or a sports activity. If your child has not been active and seems to tire quickly, encourage him or her to start out slowly (less time) and keep at it! Fifteen minutes twice a day may be enough for a start. Remember that being active can take on many different forms, and it does not have to be formal exercise. If your child gets involved with routine physical activities around the home, this can serve as a great way to get exercise and possibly earn an allowance or reward from you! Whether it's mowing the lawn, raking leaves, or washing the car, it all counts as physical activity.

Activity in the Disabled and Chronically Ill

For people with orthopedic conditions, joint pain, or musculoskeletal problems, low-impact exercise is usually the best bet. Swimming is a good low-impact form of resistance exercise. If you are in a wheelchair or unable to stand or stay on your feet for long periods without support, chair exercises may also be a good option. There are a number of chair-exercise DVDs available for at-home work.

Wheelchair-Bound Exercise Options

Even if you can't use your lower body, it's important to keep your upper body active and toned to get all the health benefits of regular exercise. There are plenty of exercises that can be done while sitting, including lifting light weights and using resistance bands. Speak with your doctor first to get medical clearance, and then consider seeing an exercise physiologist who can help you design a workout from your wheelchair.

Exercising for the Elderly

Staying active is particularly important as you grow older. Aging is associated with increased insulin resistance, and it's thought that this is at least partially attributable to a loss of muscle mass. Keep on track with an active lifestyle and strength-training exercises to retain muscle mass and insulin sensitivity. It's never too late to get moving. Talk to your doctor today about an appropriate exercise program that promotes strength, balance, flexibility, and endurance.

Dealing with Obesity When Exercising

If you are extremely overweight or obese, exercise is especially important yet can present unique challenges. Comfort is an issue; certain exercises such as jogging and high-impact aerobics may simply not be feasible. Weight lies heavy on the mind as well as the body, and it's possible you may not feel mentally or emotionally prepared to join group or team exercises. The solution is to work on your own level. Don't try step aerobics just yet. Contact your local YMCA or community center to see if there's a plus-size exercise program available. And always check with your doctor before starting a new fitness routine. A referral to an exercise physiologist may be appropriate, particularly if you have other health problems. It may be easier said than done, but don't feel self-conscious. If you feel uncomfortable amid all the spandex and ripped abs at the local health club, then don't torture yourself—find an environment that you feel better in. Try a walking program, either outside or at home on a treadmill. Buddy up with a friend and motivate each other to reach workout goals. Exercise should make you feel good about yourself. Every step you take is a step toward a healthier you.

Keeping It in Perspective

Many people with prediabetes/diabetes start exercising for the sole purpose of losing weight. When the pounds don't drop as quickly or as completely as they'd like, some of these people get discouraged and give up. If you take away any message about exercise and prediabetes, let it be this:

even if you don't lose weight, your investment in exercise is still paying off in reduced heart disease risk and better blood sugar control. Also, remember, exercise builds muscle, which weighs more than fat. If your clothes fit better, but the pounds don't melt off as much as you'd hoped—you are still ahead of the game. And exercise simply makes you feel better, both physically and mentally. Your energy level will rise, and the endorphins released by your brain during exercise will boost your sense of well-being and may help fight prediabetes-related depression. Don't give up before you really get started. You owe it to yourself to keep going.

Slow and Steady Wins the Race

Once you have had success with starting and maintaining your exercise, branch out and find new ways to get exercise and keep it interesting. Varying the routine helps to keep you from getting bored, and it challenges your body in different ways. An exercise plan of walking can be augmented by including strength training and stretching. Your exercise program should be one that you can maintain for life. Make sensible decisions about what you can and will change to increase your activity level. You may realize some of the benefits of exercise early on, but long-lasting results come about with consistency. Think of your exercise program as a work in progress that you are constantly improving and finding new ways to derive health benefits and enjoyment from. Slow, steady progress will help you achieve your goals, and you will realize how worthwhile your efforts have been.

Here are some habits that will integrate exercise into your daily routine.

21. Schedule Activity Into Your Calendar

These days everyone is *so* busy, and multitasking is the new norm. It can be easy to get caught up in other things and lose out on time for exercise, which is important for keeping your blood sugar and weight in check. You really need to plan for and take time out to do regular exercise.

Tips to Make the Habit Stick

- Make regular activity a priority by blocking out time in your day for exercise—consider it an appointment that you cannot miss.
- If you have a pretty regular schedule, you may find a particular time during the day that works best for you to get into a good routine.
- If your schedule is varied and changes frequently, you may want to plan your activity week by week, taking a look at your schedule in advance and penciling it in when you see open times.
- Use calendar reminders and alarms to help you remember.

22. Get Sporty with Your Exercise Routine

Instead of just watching sports, get out there and play some! Sports are a great way to add variety and healthy competition to your exercise routine. Even when you don't feel much like exercising, your commitment to other team members may get you moving, and it's a great way to meet new friends and keep up a regular exercise plan to help control your prediabetes.

Tips to Make the Habit Stick

- Join an adult beginner team, such as a local softball or soccer league.
- Try a biking group or running club.
- Participate in a tennis club.

23. Keep Your Kids Active

There are plenty of things your child or teen can do to become active every day to help with blood sugars and weight. Talk with your child about what type of activities he or she thinks might be fun or interesting to try. If other family members or friends participate in the activity too, your child will be more willing to go along. It is more fun to be active with others. Encourage children to be active in a variety of fun and easy ways.

Tips to Make the Habit Stick

- Think about programs offered at the YMCA, YWCA, or other community groups that offer physical activity.
- Offer to go for a walk or bike ride with your child after dinner.
- Suggest trying a new activity such as skateboarding, bowling, or an after-school sports league activity, which might be appealing.
- Even walking to and from school is a great way to start getting more active. Get an inexpensive pedometer for your child, so she can count daily activity steps and work toward achieving 10,000 steps a day. Some studies suggest that 10,000 steps a day is about the right number of steps to be considered exercise. When you use a pedometer to figure out how many steps you take every day, you may be surprised to learn that your child is not moving nearly enough.

24. Get Walking

For most people, walking is a good place to begin an exercise program because it is easy and requires no special equipment other than a pair of good walking shoes or sneakers. Brisk walking is considered an aerobic exercise, which means your body is using oxygen. Aerobic exercise increases your heart rate and burns calories to help with weight and blood sugars. Walking in this manner is considered an effective type of exercise for weight loss. And any extra walking you do throughout the day also adds up, so try walking as a good start to your exercise plan.

Tips to Make the Habit Stick

- If you choose to walk and have not exercised in a long time, you may need to begin by walking at a moderate pace. Walking about three times a week for a period of ten to fifteen minutes can help ease you into a routine.
- As you become stronger and gain more endurance, gradually increase your walking time by five minutes every one to two weeks, until you are able to walk for a full thirty minutes. Once you are comfortable walking for thirty minutes, increase your frequency to four or five times weekly, and gradually pick up the pace to a brisk walk.

25. Invest in a Pedometer

An excellent way to stay motivated and track your progress with walking is to use a pedometer. A pedometer is a small, inexpensive device that counts the number of steps you take in the course of a day. Using a pedometer can be helpful to ensure that you are getting in your daily steps to promote control of your prediabetes.

Tips to Make the Habit Stick

- A pedometer is usually clipped to your belt or waistband and, if worn from the beginning to the end of your day, will count each step that you take.
- You can determine your daily step total by wearing the pedometer for three consecutive full days, then dividing the step total by three. Once you know the average steps you take per day, you can set small goals for yourself to increase the total number of steps you take every day.

26. Liven Up Exercise with Your Own Soundtrack

Keep your workout interesting with some audio entertainment! There is such a variety of music and other forms of audio these days to choose from to help you stay moving.

Tips to Make the Habit Stick

- Listen to the radio or, better yet, make your own custom playlist to enjoy your favorite tunes while working out. This is a great way to get you moving to the beat while promoting weight and blood sugar management.
- Another option is to exercise your mind as well as your body with an audiobook.
- Try exercising without the iPod for once and enjoy the sounds of nature and the neighborhood.

27. Don't Just Sit There

Research has shown that avoiding prolonged periods of sitting may help prevent type 2 diabetes for those at risk and may help blood sugar control in those already diagnosed with type 2 diabetes. Move around as often as possible.

Tips to Make the Habit Stick

• Try to avoid sitting for longer than thirty–sixty minutes. Stand up, take a bathroom break, go get a glass of water, take a short walk, or do a few stretches to reenergize and stay healthy.

• Setting a timer can be helpful to remind you to take breaks from sitting at regular intervals.

28. Break It Up

If you don't have a full thirty–sixty-minute block in your day to work out, try working in ten minutes of activity several times a day, and the benefits will add up. There are many ways you can add in a little bit of activity to your day without making huge demands on your schedule. And, putting activity into a busy day by doing just ten minutes here and there will add up to help control your prediabetes.

Tips to Make the Habit Stick

- Find opportunities to walk by arriving at your destination early, parking farther away, and then walking for ten minutes.
- Take the stairs whenever you can and do this several times during the day. Avoid elevators.
- Go for a ten-minute walk after lunch or dinner.
- Spend ten minutes at the beginning and end of each day doing a few resistance and stretching exercises. It's healthy and will make you feel good about the start of your day.

29. Make Exercise a Chore, Literally

You may not realize it, but many routine household activities such as cleaning, vacuuming, carrying groceries, gardening, and yard work are all forms of physical activity that can help bring down blood sugars and burn calories. Include this type of activity in your daily routine.

Tips to Make the Habit Stick

- Use your daily chore list as a way to get in more activity and keep a clean house while you are at it.
- Accomplish two things at once by cleaning and working out at the same time.
- Keep in mind there are many household chores, and you can burn calories by doing them for as little as half an hour. Here are some examples of different chores and the calories they burn per thirty minutes:

  - Sweeping, washing dishes, laundry, and dusting = "light" activity/ 90–100 calories
  - Gardening, mowing the lawn, raking leaves, scrubbing floors, vacuuming, washing cars, washing windows, carrying out trash, shoveling snow/dirt = "moderate" activity/130–200 calories

30. Pair Up with an Exercise Buddy, or Two or Three...

Working out with a friend, family member, or colleague helps keep activity fun and social and is a great motivator to help you stick to your exercise plan to control prediabetes. It requires you to plan ahead to schedule your activity, and your partner can hold you accountable to complete it. Plus, you will be amazed at how fast the time goes by during your workout when you are walking and talking with a friend. Being able to support one another is a positive feeling. The more exercise buddies, the merrier to keep things upbeat. Work on working out with others.

Tips to Make the Habit Stick

- Find different buddies to do a variety of activities with such as biking, tennis, walking, and so on.
- Many communities have exercise groups for running, biking, etc., so you can always research that as an additional, great option.
- Some people find a regular session with a certified personal trainer works well as a "buddy" who can also provide useful instruction. If it is within your budget, give it a shot.

31. Don't Take Time-Outs During Travel

It may be tempting to let your commitment to exercise slide if you go on vacation or a work trip, but with a little extra effort and planning you can remain active even when away from home and out of your usual routine. Be sure to factor in activity during your vacation; don't leave it out—remember, it is key to controlling your prediabetes.

Tips to Make the Habit Stick

- If you are traveling by air, budget extra time to do a few minutes of walking in the airport and to your gate before your flight.

- Have a long drive ahead? Plan to stop a few times to take a ten-minute walk after a bathroom break or a meal.

- When at your destination, take advantage of the hotel gym in the morning or before dinner. Another fun option is to explore your new surroundings with a brisk walk.

- Hectic work trips may require extra planning to work activity in, such as getting up twenty to thirty minutes earlier to hit the gym or go out for a jog. Bring along a trusty workout DVD that you can do in your room when it is convenient. Walk to dinner, take the stairs instead of the elevator, and move around during lunch and other break times.

- If you are lucky enough to be on vacation, attempt to plan a fun getaway with fitness in mind. Water activities such as swimming, snorkeling, and kayaking are great in warm climates. A bike ride, hike, or walking tour would be great during moderate temperatures. Winter activities like skiing, snowshoeing, ice-skating, and sledding are a superfun way to get your exercise in a colder atmosphere.

32. Challenge Yourself by Setting Personal Exercise Goals

Setting small, realistic, and positive goals can be a way to keep active and step up your activity levels incrementally. Setting daily, weekly, and monthly goals can help you stay on track and continue to challenge yourself to stay active and continually improve your fitness level that is so important to managing your prediabetes. Break your goals into small steps to climb the fitness ladder to success.

Tips to Make the Habit Stick

- If you have never exercised before and have been given the go-ahead by your doctor, a small goal of five or ten minutes per day is an example of a great start.
- If you are already in the habit of exercising, set a goal of adding an additional five minutes to your session or adding an extra session into your week.
- To increase variety, make it a goal to try one new activity per month to enhance your fitness routine.

33. Take Advantage of Technology

There is a plethora of digital fitness tools and trackers out there these days, many of which you may find very helpful to support you in your exercise goals to help manage your prediabetes. Add digital support and monitoring to enhance your fitness routine.

Tips to Make the Habit Stick

- Do some research on the Internet and mobile app stores to find a tracking app that best meets your needs. Options currently available range from food and activity trackers, to wearable devices to track heart rate/sleep habits/steps, to online workouts and support communities. Some technologies can even send data to your healthcare team for more detailed monitoring.
- See Appendix C at the end of the book for some great tracker suggestions.

34. Make Activity a Family Affair

Make plans with your family to do something active together at least once a week. That way you get to spend quality time with each other and get some exercise too. Being active as a family sets a good example for your children to continue during their lives, and it helps to keep your weight and blood sugars under control while you're at it. Go ahead and get fit, family-style!

Tips to Make the Habit Stick

- Try simple activities like a family bike ride, walk/hike, or going to the park to play basketball or kick a soccer ball around. These activities don't cost anything, and you will get the added benefit of some physical activity.
- You don't have to go far to get in family fitness; even hula hooping in the garage together or having a dance party in the living room count toward exercise.
- Look online for maps of local walking trails. It can be a great way to stay in touch with nature while getting some good cardio.

35. Try an Exercise Class

Enrolling in a class at your local gym, fitness center, or recreation center is a great way to try something new, meet others, and get some helpful guidance from an instructor. Incorporate fitness classes to help add variety into your exercise routine to improve your blood sugars and manage weight.

Tips to Make the Habit Stick

- Take advantage of all your options. There are so many to choose from these days, such as yoga, Pilates, aerobics, CrossFit, kickboxing, sculpting, water aerobics...you name it!

- When you find a class you like, check and see if the gym or fitness center offers specials or the option to pay for a block of classes ahead of time. Doing this will often get you a small discount, and it helps hold you accountable to show up for multiple sessions in the future.

- Many classes incorporate weights or exercises using your own body weight, which can be a great way to get your resistance training under the observation of a skilled instructor.

- Intimidated by the thought of doing a class in public? Investigate fitness workouts via DVD or streamed online. You can try them in the comfort of your own home.

36. Take Up Exercise As a Hobby or As a Way to Volunteer

You may not realize it, but there are many fun hobbies that are actually very active. There are many opportunities to learn something new or even help others while you exercise.

Tips to Make the Habit Stick

- Try a fun new hobby such as dancing, bowling, golfing, wood-working, or badminton, to name just a few.
- Use volunteer work as a way to help out the community and get active at the same time. Helping as a crossing guard, dog walking at a shelter, helping build housing for the needy, being part of a walkathon or fun run for charity, coaching a local kids' team, or helping organize items at a food pantry or donation center will get you moving to help with your prediabetes. At the same time, you're doing good for your community.

37. Be Safe with Your Exercise Routine

While physical activity can be a great thing for your health, make sure to take the proper precautions so that your workouts are safe and you can avoid injury or exhaustion. Make safety a priority along with regular activity as part of your prediabetes action plan.

Tips to Make the Habit Stick

- Consult with your doctor to obtain medical approval before beginning an exercise program.

- Warm up and stretch your muscles for at least five minutes before beginning a workout and do a five-minute cooldown at the end as well.

- Avoid exercising outside in extreme temperatures (superhot or very cold) or consider changing your workout to indoors in these temperatures.

- Exercise at an intensity that feels moderate and comfortable; don't overdo it.

- Wear breathable, comfortable clothing and sturdy footwear during workouts.

- Hydrate adequately before, during, and after your workout.

- If you're working with weights, make sure you get some initial instruction about proper form and positioning from an experienced trainer.

- Stop activity if you feel any pain, dizziness, difficulty breathing, or chest pain and let your doctor know if you have experienced any of these symptoms during exercise.

38. Consider Adopting a Furry Friend

You would be amazed at how a pet can change your life and your fitness level for the better. Not to mention research has shown that pets can be great for your mood and emotional support, which is a win-win for helping control your prediabetes. Consider a companion pet that will encourage you to be out and about!

Tips to Make the Habit Stick

- Think about getting a dog to get you out there moving since you will now have a built-in fitness buddy for walks, jogs, or playing around at the park.
- Use the responsibility you have for your pet to motivate you to exercise more than once per day. Realize that taking short walks, multiple times a day will add up.

39. Don't Forget to Hydrate and Fuel Your Workouts

Having the proper hydration and adequate fuel can make a big difference in your workout performance, but you don't need to overdo it either. Fuel and hydrate yourself appropriately before fitness to maximize your workout for blood sugar and weight control.

Tips to Make the Habit Stick

- For liquids, a general guideline is to drink two cups of fluid within two hours of starting exercise and to drink at least ½ cup of fluid every fifteen minutes during exercise. After your workout, drink two to three cups for every pound of fluid lost. Beware of sugary sports drinks; there is no need for them if you are exercising for sixty minutes or less—water will be just fine.

- If you have worked up to doing more intense and longer endurance exercise, then you may require some carbohydrates and electrolytes, and it would be a good idea to consult with a dietitian to create a plan.

- Don't run on empty; make sure you have eaten a snack or meal within one to two hours before your workout. Ideally, eat something with a bit of carbohydrate and some protein, such as ½ banana or rice cake with 1 tablespoon of peanut butter or a light yogurt, for example.

40. Know Your Reps During Resistance

Using resistance training with varied and increasing repetitions and sets can help you get stronger, not to mention help control your prediabetes. It is important to become familiar with the amount of repetitions and sets of various exercises that should be completed to get the maximum benefits from your routine in a safe way.

Tips to Make the Habit Stick

- Consulting with a certified trainer can take the guesswork out of resistance training, if you have been approved to start strength training by your physician.
- When doing resistance training with weights or bands, your initial goal should be to try to complete one to two sets of 10–15 repetitions per set. Get to where you are feeling near fatigue in that muscle when done.
- As you get stronger you can progress by using gradually heavier weights/resistance to where you can complete at least 8–10 repetitions per set. You can follow the increase in weight/resistance by increasing the number of sets (for example, instead of doing 1–2 sets of repetitions, try 2–3 sets).
- If you have a history of joint/muscle issues or other health limitations, start with just one set of 10–15 repetitions with a lighter weight, then progress to 15–20 repetitions before increasing the number of sets.

Chapter 6

Lose It! Manage Your Weight for Life

THERE IS DEFINITELY a significant link between excess weight and blood sugar control. Let's review the startling statistics (mentioned in Chapter 2) again: more than one-third of adults (36.5 percent) in the US are obese, and the rate of childhood obesity is also skyrocketing with more than 18 percent of our nation's children classified as obese. America as a nation has been packing on the pounds for the past two decades. Eighty percent of people with type 2 diabetes are also overweight or obese. Luckily, there is very strong evidence that managing obesity can prevent and delay the progression of prediabetes to diabetes. Losing weight is one of the best ways to treat prediabetes, but it can also be very challenging.

Benefits of Weight Loss

When beginning your weight loss journey, it can be very helpful and motivating to learn about all the health benefits of shedding excess pounds. Losing weight makes a big difference in your body's ability to control blood sugar. The Diabetes Prevention Program (DPP) proved that even modest weight loss can prevent or delay the onset of type 2 diabetes in overweight at-risk adults.

Weight and Insulin Resistance

Precisely how excess fat promotes insulin resistance isn't yet entirely clear, but it is thought that stored fat releases certain proteins and/or enzymes that act on muscle and liver cells to impair the way they "read" insulin signals to process glucose. In addition, research has found that the "apple-shaped" body (central abdominal obesity) associated with insulin resistance and type 2 diabetes contains fat with unique properties. Specifically, this type of visceral abdominal fat sheds more free fatty acids, which can elevate triglyceride levels, and is associated with higher insulin levels that promote further fat storage. Paring down abdominal fat will have the double benefit of both increasing insulin sensitivity and decreasing triglyceride levels in people with prediabetes and type 2 diabetes.

Other Health Benefits of Weight Loss

In addition to keeping your prediabetes in check, there are numerous other health benefits to losing weight (even just 5–10 percent of your body weight) including:

- Improved mobility and less stress on your joints, lowered risk of osteoarthritis

- Greater sense of well-being, more energy, improved mood, and positive self-image
- Lowered risk of many chronic diseases like some types of cancer, cardiovascular disease, and diabetes
- Decreased levels of inflammation in the body, lower blood pressure, and lower cholesterol
- Better sleep, and in those with sleep apnea (a sleep disorder commonly diagnosed in those with excess weight) improvements and sometimes resolution of the condition

Reducing Calories, One of the Cornerstones of Weight Loss

A calorie (a.k.a. kilocalorie) is scientifically defined as the amount of energy required to raise the temperature of 1 gram of water by 1 degree Celsius. To put this in layperson's terms, a calorie is basically a unit of energy your body uses as fuel. The three main macronutrients, or sources of calories, are carbohydrates, proteins, and fats. Carbohydrates and proteins each provide 4 calories per gram, whereas fats provide more than double that at 9 calories per gram. In addition, alcohol provides 7 calories per gram. Foods tend to be mixtures of carbs, protein, and fats so each food has its unique calorie value that you will find on nutrition labels and in food charts. Keep in mind that when you are on a particular calorie budget for weight loss, you want to consume foods that are nutrient dense, meaning they have the most nutrients, like healthy carbs, proteins, fats, fiber, vitamins, and minerals for the lowest number of calories they contain. For example, a mixed vegetable salad with grilled chicken breast would be high in protein, fiber, vitamins, and minerals all at a lower calorie cost. In comparison, a piece of chocolate cake would be sky-high in calories, sugar, and fat yet would lack high-fiber carbs and contain very little key nutrients.

What Should Your Caloric Intake Be?

Your ideal calorie intake is based on your activity level, gender, age, and other factors. Reducing calorie intake is one component of an effective weight-reduction program, so it is also an important consideration in the dietary management of prediabetes.

Very Low-Calorie Diets?

The ADA 2018 *Standards of Care* states, "To achieve weight loss of > 5% in the short-term (3-month) interventions that use very low-calorie diets (≤800 kcal/day) and total meal replacements may be prescribed for carefully selected patients by trained practitioners in medical care settings with close medical monitoring. To maintain weight loss, such programs must incorporate long-term comprehensive weight maintenance counseling." Generally, diets under 1,200 calories per day are not recommended for the long term and require medical supervision while they are undertaken.

The estimated amounts of daily calorie intake based on gender, age, and activity levels from the US Department of Agriculture's 2015–2020 *Dietary Guidelines for Americans* can be found at: https://health.gov/dietaryguidelines/2015/guidelines/appendix-2/. These are general guidelines for weight maintenance, not weight loss. The ADA suggests a lifestyle program with a diet approach of reduced calories (500 to 750 fewer calories than the USDA guidelines listed for weight maintenance) or approximately 1,200–1,500 calories a day for women and 1,500–1,800 calories a day for men.

There is no single suggested diet composition for everyone. Diets should be individualized to achieve lower calorie levels, but they may differ in protein, carbohydrate, and fat content. The guidelines just listed are general, so an important part of this approach involves education and support via meeting with a registered dietitian regularly. You can work together to decide upon your calorie goal and get an individualized meal plan that will be helpful to your efforts to lose weight. You will want to focus on making changes for the long term that you can live with and that will allow you to eat a variety of foods you enjoy. Beware of fad diets that promise quick fixes, are overly restrictive, and cut out key nutrients, because their success is often not scientifically proven.

The Low-Carb Conundrum

Low-carb diets are the subject of heated debate in the diabetes community. At first glance, the issue seems cut-and-dried. Carbohydrates cause blood sugar to rise, so wouldn't a low-carb diet automatically be beneficial for someone with diabetes? But low-carb also goes against everything the USDA and nutritionists have been saying for the past several decades— that the vast majority of your calories (45–65 percent) should come from carbohydrates.

The Pros and Cons of a Low-Carbohydrate Diet

It's an undisputed fact that dietary carbohydrates increase blood sugar levels. Minimize your carb intake, and you'll minimize increases in blood glucose. So, a low-carb diet appears to have a logical, though still disputed, place in diabetes management. But what about low-carb for weight loss? In a nutshell, low-carb proponents blame weight gain on high insulin levels, which can promote fat storage. Since insulin release is triggered by dietary carbohydrates, the reasoning is that too many carbs mean too much glucose, which in turn leads to high levels of circulating insulin (hyperinsulinemia), which causes fat storage and weight gain.

This hyperinsulinemia can also lead to inflammation in the body that can worsen insulin resistance over time. The ADA does not endorse low-carb plans for long-term diabetes control, saying that the high-fat and high-protein content in these diets can be dangerous for people with diabetes who are already at risk for coronary artery disease.

Net Carbs

Clients sometimes say to me, "I keep seeing 'net carbs' on different foods at the grocery store. What does that mean?"

"Net carbs" and "effective carbs" are marketing terms coined by food manufacturers. In theory, "net carbs" are those that impact blood sugar. That means that the manufacturer has subtracted carbs from ingredients like sugar alcohols, glycerin, and fiber from the total carbohydrate grams. Proceed with caution and test your blood sugar before and after eating to see if that "net carb" number really works for you.

The other issue with low-carb diets is their high-protein content, which can be tough on the kidneys of people who have advanced kidney disease. Nonetheless, many people swear by such programs—saying that a low-carb diet has given them their blood sugar control back.

Most successful low-carb plans require dieters to pay attention to calories as well as carbs; too much fat can add too many calories to your diet, and without calorie reduction, weight loss simply won't occur. If you do decide to give low-carb dieting a try, discuss it with your doctor first, and then work with your registered dietitian on a customized plan for you.

The Research on Low-Carb

In 2003, *The New England Journal of Medicine* published two important controlled clinical trials that put low-carb diets to the test among people with significant weight and health problems. One study found that obese participants with diabetes who were restricted to 30 grams of carbs daily achieved greater weight loss, maintained better glucose control, and cut triglyceride levels more than their counterparts who were put on a low-fat diet. The second trial had a smaller study population but came to similar conclusions. However, the authors also concluded that the difference in the health benefits between low-fat and low-carb became insignificant after the first six months.

Low-Carb Diets Are Potentially Effective

In 2008, the American Diabetes Association issued its first-ever formal clinical recognition of the potential benefit of low-carb dieting, stating in its nutrition guidelines that low-carb diets "may be effective in the short term" (i.e., up to two years) for weight loss.

Subsequent trials have also revealed weight loss and health benefits to low-carb eating. One of these was the *A to Z Weight Loss Study*, which put four popular weight-loss diets—Atkins, Ornish, LEARN, and the Zone—in a head-to-head competition. Results published in *The Journal of the American Medical Association* found that twelve months into the study, those study subjects on the low-carb Atkins program had lost the most weight and achieved the biggest health benefits (in terms of improved cholesterol profiles and lower fasting insulin and glucose levels), as compared to those on the higher-carb alternative diets. However, a meta-analysis of studies of low-carb versus low-fat diets for weight loss published in the *Archives of Internal Medicine* concluded that while low-carb diets were at least as effective as low-fat diets for weight loss, they were associated with unfavorable changes in total and LDL (bad) cholesterol levels. On a more positive note, the study also found that low-carb dieting was associated with favorable changes in triglyceride and HDL (good) cholesterol levels. Further long-term, large-scale trials are needed to analyze the risks and potential pluses of a low-carb diet in diabetes treatment. In the meantime, the bottom line is that current research does acknowledge some benefits of limiting carbohydrates for weight loss and diabetes control. If you have high LDL or total cholesterol, your doctor should monitor your cholesterol levels carefully if you choose to go on a low-carb diet.

More Than Just Calories and Diet

If you are overweight and have prediabetes, keep in mind that even modest weight loss can decrease insulin resistance and improve control. But calorie reduction alone as a weight-loss strategy rarely leads to long-term weight control. The three main components of a sound weight-loss program include eating a healthy diet (described in Chapter 4) that is calorie controlled, regular activity (reviewed in Chapter 5), and behavior modification, which will be discussed in more detail next.

Behavior Modification

Behavior modification can make all the difference between knowing what to do and actually doing it and remaining successful when it comes to weight loss. Some main principles of behavior modification for weight management include:

Self-Monitoring

Keeping a food journal can be very helpful in your weight-loss journey. Keeping a diary of your weight-loss progress can help you become familiar with the things that trigger weight gain and slip-ups for you and can make you much less likely to fall prey to them the next time around. It also provides detailed information for your dietitian and doctor to use when creating treatment plans.

Goal Setting and Shaping

Deciding upon and setting small goals in the short term can help set you up for long-term success. Meeting your goals and building on them incrementally can be a great motivator to continue to move forward.

Stimulus Control

Identifying triggers that create barriers and setbacks to achieving your weight-loss goals is key so that you can prevent them and correct them.

Stress Management

Stress, depression, and mood issues can create large roadblocks to achieving your goals. It is important to find techniques to manage stress and also to identify or deal with mood disorders that you may be experiencing and seek medical help if needed.

Social Support

It is tough to lose weight all on your own. Creating a support network of family, friends, medical professionals, and even support groups can help give you that extra encouragement you need as well as help with problem-solving and staying positive through your challenges.

Some of these techniques can be self-taught, but you will find that meeting with a dietitian and behavior therapist will be necessary to help you learn and incorporate these behavior modification principles. Having that extra guidance and professional support on a regular basis can make all the difference.

Emotional Eating

Emotional eating is defined as eating in response to emotional triggers such as stress or negative emotions. It can occur in response to dieting or independently due to other factors. There are many suggested mechanisms for why emotional eating occurs, ranging from history of emotional trauma, negative life events, sleep deprivation, subtypes of depression, confusion of internal states of hunger and satiety, and physiological symptoms associated with emotions or insufficient emotional regulation abilities in the body. Emotional eating is often used as a dysfunctional way to cope with negative feelings or as a distraction to try to avoid them. During an emotional eating episode, it is common to turn to comfort foods high in sugar, salt, and fat, which leads to feelings of guilt. This guilt, in turn, triggers more emotional eating, and it becomes an unhealthy cycle.

If you think that you may have problems with emotional eating, especially if it happens repeatedly and is out of control, it is important to get help. The best thing you can do is be honest with yourself that there is a problem. There is no shame in admitting you're emotionally eating and trying to get better. Working with a behavioral therapist and dietitian can help you identify triggers, process your feelings, develop positive nonfood coping mechanisms, and ensure that you have a meal plan that is not too strict. Such a meal plan can lead to feelings of deprivation, which may put you at risk for emotional eating to begin with.

The Signs of Emotional Eating

Common signs of emotional eating behavior are sudden onset of an intense need to eat (namely unhealthy foods), mindless eating of often large quantities of food, not feeling satisfied despite eating a lot of calories, and feeling guilt or shame after an episode of emotional eating.

Other Treatments for Weight Loss: Medications

When diet and exercise just aren't doing the job, there are other options. There are a variety of medications approved by the FDA for both short- and long-term weight loss. Lomaira (phentermine) is approved for very short-term use (a few weeks) when used with additional modifications. Five medications for long-term use have been approved by the FDA currently in patients with a BMI greater than or equal to 27 who also have one or more obesity-associated comorbid conditions (such as type 2 diabetes, hypertension, and elevated cholesterol) and in patients with a BMI greater than or equal to 30 who have expressed motivation to lose weight. They include: Xenical or Alli (orlistat), BELVIQ (lorcaserin), Qsymia (phentermine plus topiramate), CONTRAVE (naltrexone plus bupropion), and Saxenda (liraglutide).

These medications all have different mechanisms of action and are used to help patients gain improved adherence to low-calorie diets in the setting of a lifestyle modification that includes exercise. An average weight loss of 2.5–5.9 kilograms (5.5–12.9 pounds) in a year can be expected with these medications. They all have potential side effects, so you should only use them under a doctor's care with careful assessment of risks versus benefits. If you're interested in learning more, talk to your doctor to see if any of these would be right for you.

Metabolic Surgery

Finally, for severely obese people who have progressed to type 2 diabetes and who have been unable to lose weight using traditional means, gastric bypass or reduction surgery, also called metabolic surgery, may be an option. Only patients with a BMI greater or equal to 35–40 are typically considered for metabolic surgery.

A number of different types of bariatric surgery are available, including adjustable gastric banding, vertical banded gastroplasty, Roux-en-Y gastric bypass, and biliopancreatic diversion (with or without a duodenal switch). The first two of these are restrictive surgeries that work by closing off the majority of the stomach to the digestive process, leaving only a small section to digest food. The latter two are bypass (or malabsorptive) operations, which reroute the digestive flow past part or all of the small intestine to minimize the number of calories that can be absorbed.

Laparoscopic adjustable banding (also called lap banding) is the most common type of bariatric surgical procedure. As with traditional adjustable gastric banding, a portion of the stomach is banded off with a device that can be inflated or deflated to change the size of the stomach pouch as required. However, lap banding uses a minimally invasive laparoscopic procedure that involves small incisions and the use of surgical cameras to position the band. This technique minimizes both recovery time and the risk of complications (as compared to traditional bariatric surgery).

It is important to choose a metabolic surgery center that is well experienced, one in which you will have access to a multidisciplinary team of doctors, nurses, dietitians, and behavioral therapists who will provide quality care. Metabolic surgery carries the same risks of infection and hemorrhage as any major surgery, plus a high rate of related complications; up to 20 percent of people who have bariatric surgery have to undergo follow-up operations to fix abdominal hernias or other problems. Gallstones are also a risk because of the rapid weight loss that occurs following the operation. Because some types of surgery bypass the small intestine, where a great deal of nutrient absorption takes place, approximately 30 percent of patients end up with deficiencies of certain vitamins and minerals (a condition that can usually be corrected with supplements). If you undergo this type of procedure, you'll require long-term nutritional monitoring. In addition, the ADA recommends that people considering metabolic surgery should receive a comprehensive mental health evaluation and that surgery should not be performed on patients with histories of mental health conditions until these conditions have been fully addressed. Patients who have metabolic surgery should be continually evaluated to assess the need for ongoing mental healthcare to help them adjust to medical and mental health changes after surgery.

Recent research shows that certain bariatric surgeries improve blood sugar control independently of the weight loss they facilitate. In other words, blood sugar improvements occur post-surgery, before significant weight loss has occurred. While scientists are still researching the mechanisms behind this, they believe it is related to the changes in levels of gut hormones that gastric bypass and banding trigger.

Keeping the Weight Off

Even after losing weight via lifestyle changes, medication, and/or surgery, weight maintenance will be a lifelong challenge. Sometimes you can't control the situations that put the pounds back on. Illness or injury can hamper your exercise efforts or required drug therapy may promote weight gain. When health conditions cause weight gain, sometimes the only thing you can do is wait it out and get back on your program when things resolve.

You can avoid slipping back into old habits like emotional eating, exercise avoidance, or plain old procrastination. In fact, having prediabetes may make it easier for you to stay on track, because you have to pay attention to your body by default. When you do stumble—and chances are that you will—remember that it isn't the end of the world. You're simply learning another lesson about yourself and your health that will benefit your emotional management of prediabetes in the long run. Now let's talk about some great healthy habits to help lose weight and keep it off in the long term.

41. Don't Enter Blindly

Make a plan. It can be difficult to decipher all the information about weight loss out there. This book is a great start to point you in the right direction, that's for sure. But it is also important to sync up with your medical team and a dietitian to develop a specific, individualized weight-loss program that incorporates a meal plan, physical activity, and behavior modification for your prediabetes. Seek out support from your medical team to create a comprehensive and personalized plan for weight loss.

Tips to Make the Habit Stick

- Plan regular visits with your team to set goals, weigh in, evaluate progress, and help deal with setbacks.
- Come prepared to medical or dietitian visits with a list of questions and issues and a food diary to maximize your time together and help them help you.
- Don't be afraid to speak up if you have concerns. The more you share, the better, so that your team can work with you to assist you in succeeding.

42. Set Realistic Expectations

Expecting that you will lose weight quickly is not realistic, and rapid weight loss will not be long-lasting. Losing one half to one pound a week over time will go much further in helping you achieve results. Realize that any weight loss is a good thing in the end.

Tips to Make the Habit Stick

- Instead of focusing on a specific weight number on the scale, use positive observations to stay on track. Clothing that fits better or an increased energy level are good ways to gauge your progress.
- Keep things in perspective and remind yourself that whatever amount of weight you lose will be of benefit to your blood sugar control and overall health.

43. Choose a Meal Plan That Includes Regular Meals Plus Snacks

It is important to fuel yourself adequately throughout the day. Excess hunger can lead to overeating, not to mention making you feel downright cranky, and it can work against your blood sugar/weight goals. Follow a meal plan that, in addition to your regular meals, allows you to snack at planned times during the day.

Tips to Make the Habit Stick

- Eat balanced meals using the plate method previously discussed (¼ of your plate protein + ¼ plate of starchy foods, and the other ½ filled with non-starchy vegetables). Add two or three sensible snacks in between that include a source of protein or healthy fat, along with a high fiber carbohydrate.

- Wash your meals down with plenty of low-calorie fluids, and you are setting yourself up for success.

- Look at your schedule in advance to plan times that you can eat, especially during weeks that are busy or when you are traveling.

- Set alarms or timers to remind yourself to eat meals and snacks and drink water so you don't get caught up in the chaos of a hectic day and forget to eat and drink.

44. Plan to Treat Yourself Once in a While

Of course, it is difficult (and for most, pretty impossible) to never eat the foods you love. If you decide never to eat a particular food, you may become obsessed with it and end up overeating it when given the opportunity. Lifelong healthy eating is about choices and finding a way to balance all the foods that you enjoy within reason as far as your prediabetes plan is concerned.

Tips to Make the Habit Stick

- Don't deprive yourself of the foods you love; instead give yourself permission to have the food during a special occasion or celebration. Develop strategies ahead of time to work them into your meal plan occasionally. A dietitian can help work with you on this challenge.
- Find a way to balance the problem food in a healthy way by not restricting it but rather reserving it for a certain time when you are free to really enjoy it.
- Plan to "cheat" by eating lighter at meals before and after your splurge.
- When treating yourself, remember it is all about portion control. Have a smaller serving of your favorite food as part of a healthy meal that also includes plenty of vegetables and protein (that helps keep you full) in order to avoid overdoing it.

45. Stock Your Pantry and Fridge with the Right Foods

Having healthy alternatives available when you are hungry encourages adherence to your meal plan, whereas having high-calorie foods, snacks, and desserts invites temptation. Relying on willpower to stop you from eating irresistible foods will not work if you are faced with these food choices every day. In fact, willpower should not be one of your ongoing strategies to improve your eating habits. Instead, keep yourself in check by stocking your pantry and fridge with healthy choices.

Tips to Make the Habit Stick

- Make over your pantry by shopping according to a list of foods that fit your meal plan and throw out or give away any foods that are not on your prediabetes meal plan. Remove your problem foods from the house on a regular basis, and you will begin to move away from consuming these foods. Try to consume your treats when you are out so they are not in the house to tempt you for repeat consumption.

- Keep your food environment safer by keeping healthier food and snack alternatives available at all times. Precut veggies and fruit for snacking and meals are helpful to keep on hand as well as high-protein foods like cooked chicken, peanut butter, hard-boiled eggs, and precooked beans. Having plenty of healthy food choices ready to eat helps you avoid the pitfalls of eating too many empty-calorie foods that get in the way of weight loss or managing your prediabetes. Check Appendix A at the end of this book for some helpful grocery list suggestions.

46. Eat Mindfully

We are all so busy these days it is too easy to gobble down a meal without knowing how much we've eaten. Make time to focus on your food and enjoy it by taking time out to eat without distractions, otherwise it is easy to lose track and decrease the positive control you can have over your eating habits.

Tips to Make the Habit Stick

- Try taking time to really enjoy your food and slow down eating by putting your fork down between bites. Take some time to sit down and have meals and snacks. It is better for your digestion not to rush as well.

- Eat away from the television and other distractions that make it too easy to gobble up twice as much as you intended.

- Focus on how the food tastes and its different textures and pay attention to when you feel full; not only will you get more satisfaction from eating but you will keep portions in check, as well as your weight and blood sugars.

- If you have family, sit down and eat with them at the dining table. Spend the meal talking and interacting with one another. It will improve your digestion.

47. Scale Back the Weighing

Don't weigh yourself obsessively. Remember, weight loss is not a quick process. Once a week—at the same time of day—is all you need to monitor your progress. Set a regular time to weigh yourself weekly.

Tips to Make the Habit Stick

- Be consistent about when and how you weigh yourself. Weight can vary daily due to fluid shifts, hormones, the time of day you weigh in, and the clothing you're wearing. It is best to weigh yourself in the same manner—first thing in the morning after using the restroom and without clothes to be most accurate.

- Try to rely more on the way you feel than on the tale of the tape. If the scale tells you you're losing weight more slowly than you'd like, but you're feeling energetic and positive about your weight-loss efforts, and your blood sugars are improving, then you're heading in the right direction.

48. Exercise Regularly, No Excuses

Eating healthfully is just one part of the equation when it comes to losing weight. Even if you are sticking to your prediabetes meal plan like a champ, that does not mean you are allowed to let your activity levels slide. Chapter 5 has plenty of great tips to keep you active, but remember, don't give yourself the time or permission to procrastinate. Exercising regularly on a set schedule will help you turn this into a habit.

Tips to Make the Habit Stick

- Don't think about whether you should put off activity, just get out there and do it! Stick to your schedule, set times to exercise, get ready, and go for it. Don't give yourself the time to talk yourself out of exercising.
- Think back to how great you feel after working out and use that as a positive motivator to get moving, along with its positive effects on blood sugars and weight.

49. Eat Only When You Are Hungry

Before you reach for something in the pantry or swing open the fridge, pause to evaluate whether you are truly hungry. Take a time-out before you reach for food to decide if you really want to eat.

Tips to Make the Habit Stick

- Pause and ask yourself if you are experiencing true physical sensations of hunger or if you are experiencing something else, such as stress, boredom, or a craving for a certain food.
- If you are not truly hungry, try filling up with a glass of water, then step away from the kitchen and become engaged in a nonfood activity. Let the feeling pass until next mealtime. That way, you won't sabotage your prediabetes meal plan needlessly.
- If you're in the middle of a meal and find yourself no longer hungry, pause and wait a few minutes. If you're still not hungry at the end of that time, stop eating.

50. Avoid Eating in Bulk

A large container of food such as a bag of nuts or a tub of frozen yogurt is an open invitation to overindulge and will result in spikes in your blood sugar and weight. Even if you are stocking your kitchen with healthy foods, you still need to be aware of portions in order to stick to your calorie goal.

Tips to Make the Habit Stick

- Avoid eating straight out of the container and instead take one serving of your food out, put it on a dish, and eat it at the table.
- Use measuring cups, measuring spoons, and scales to help you portion. It is also helpful to have snacks and meals preportioned in baggies or reusable containers so you can grab and go.
- Beware of serving meals family style in large serving dishes that remain on the table and can encourage multiple self-servings. Instead portion your plate in the kitchen before you head to the table. Preportioning your foods ahead of time ensures that you don't overserve yourself.

51. Start Your Day with a Healthy Breakfast

Studies have shown that regularly eating breakfast can help with weight loss. Make time to include breakfast in your morning so you can fuel your body and mind and stave off any excess hunger, which could lead to overeating at lunch. Take a minute to fuel yourself with healthy food to start your day right.

Tips to Make the Habit Stick

- Include high-fiber carb food with some added protein to keep your blood sugar stable and help with satiety. Quick choices on the go can include a slice of toast or whole-grain waffle with 2 tablespoons of peanut butter, 1 cup of low-fat Greek yogurt or cottage cheese with ½ cup of berries or banana slices, or a stick of string cheese plus a piece of fruit.

- If you have more time to prepare a morning meal, whip up an egg white or 1-egg omelet with shredded low-fat cheese and diced veggies with a side of toast or fruit. Or try ½ cup cooked oats sprinkled with ¼ cup chopped nuts.

52. Have a Large Glass of Water Before Every Meal

Filling up on fluids before eating has been shown to be an effective weight-loss technique. A recent study conducted at the University of Birmingham compared two groups of people. In one group, participants consumed 500 milliliters of water (that's about 16 ounces or 2 cups) thirty minutes before meals. They lost 3 pounds more than the control group, which did not drink water before meals, over a twelve-week period. Those are promising results. Unless you have a medical condition that restricts fluids, there is no harm in trying some extra calorie-free hydration before meals.

Tips to Make the Habit Stick

- Sip water before every meal you eat. Start by consuming a glass of water before you even prepare your meal, so that you will already have consumed your fluids and won't forget as you start nibbling.
- When eating out, ask for water to be brought to your table before you order so you can consume your fluids in advance of your meal arriving.

53. Do Your Homework Before Eating Out

Don't let restaurant dining sabotage your prediabetes eating plan. With a little preparation you can go out and enjoy yourself but still stick to your goals. Prepare for restaurant eating by checking out the menu in advance.

Tips to Make the Habit Stick

- Investigate menu options before you even step foot in the restaurant. Most places have their menus posted online (some even include nutrition information) so you can take your time to review choices.

- If the restaurant doesn't have information posted online, then call ahead and ask questions about the menu. That way, when you are out you will not make any rushed or last-minute choices that can result in decreased adherence to your meal plan.

- Discuss with your dietitian the menu choices at your favorite restaurants. You'll get some good ideas of what to order within the scope of your meal plan. Check Appendix B for some helpful suggestions for restaurant eating.

54. Get Support

Sometimes it can be difficult to ask for help. Don't travel the road to weight loss by yourself. Instead, make it a habit to reach out to those around you for support when you need it. Let your family, friends, and colleagues know you are trying to lose weight and control your prediabetes so they can be encouraging and helpful with your efforts. Reach out to them when you are tempted to fall off the wagon or if you have had a setback. Talk things through and get back on track. Make it a priority to identify when you are beginning to feel overwhelmed. The warning signs are different for everyone. Maybe you aren't exercising as much as you once did, maybe you are becoming a bit too relaxed with your diet, maybe you feel deprived and isolated. This is the perfect time to speak up and take advantage of a support network for positive encouragement.

Tips to Make the Habit Stick

- Get your friends, family, and colleagues onboard with your eating plan so they are mindful not to bring temptations around you or into your kitchen.
- Find a buddy to share healthy recipes with and work out together to stay motivated.
- Consider a local support group through which you can meet others who are going through similar situations.
- Reach out to your medical team if you need professional guidance or help during the process; they want to help you succeed.

55. Celebrate Your Successes in a Healthy Way

If you are on the right path, meeting your goals and losing weight, be sure to acknowledge that and celebrate your success. Plan to reward yourself at regular intervals, but don't make food the focus of your rewards, as this can undo all the efforts you have been working toward to remain in control of eating and can also lead to excess calories in the long run.

Tips to Make the Habit Stick

- Try nonfood treats such as a massage, a new piece of clothing, a haircut, a new book, or an outing with friends or family.
- Don't forget to take time out to pat yourself on the back when you are successful. Be grateful and happy with your progress and use that as a positive motivator to continue to lose and maintain weight loss, as well as blood sugar control. If you feel comfortable, celebrate your successes publicly by telling others or posting on social media about your healthy habits. This can lead to extra encouragement, and you may even inspire others!

56. Add More Fiber and Healthy Volume to Your Plate

Choose to fill up on larger portions of higher-fiber, lower-calorie foods for blood sugar and weight control. Vegetables and whole-grain starches help keep you satisfied without all the calories/fat/sugar, and they have a lot of key nutrients for your body too.

Tips to Make the Habit Stick

- The best thing you can do is to always fill half your plate with non-starchy veggies—have a double portion of cooked vegetables or a salad and a cooked vegetable with your meal. Fill broth-based soup with a variety of non-starchy vegetables to add flavor and fiber. Have an entrée-sized salad composed of different lettuces and veggies with lean protein on top.
- Keep starches to small portions (a quarter of your plate) and make high-fiber choices like whole-wheat pasta, quinoa, brown rice, beans and lentils, butternut squash, peas, or sweet potato with the skin.
- Fill ¾ of your plate with high-fiber foods (½ of the plate with veggies + ¼ of the plate with a high-fiber starch).

57. Steer Clear of Weight-Loss Supplements

It may be tempting to buy the latest gimmick at the health food store or online that promises quick and easy weight loss, but don't do it. Most weight-loss supplements are not proven by sound research, are not regulated by the FDA, and may have ingredients that can interact with medications you are taking or harm your body.

Tips to Make the Habit Stick

- For some diets, a reputable vitamin and mineral supplement may be in order, so you should ask your medical team if one is required.
- Always consult with your doctor and dietitian before starting any sort of supplement.
- Skip the weight-loss supplements and make longer-lasting and safer lifestyle changes for your prediabetes instead.

58. Travel Smart and Prepared

Don't let your trip end up tripping up your weight loss and blood sugar goals. Make your trip itinerary with your health in mind. Remember that by planning ahead you can still enjoy your trip but stay in control of your prediabetes by maintaining your important eating and exercise goals.

Tips to Make the Habit Stick

- Bring along your own healthy snacks (such as baby carrots, nuts, and fruit) for your trip, drink plenty of water, and move around as often as possible.
- Try to stay in wellness-friendly hotels with healthy food options at their restaurants, that have a mini-refrigerator to store your own healthy snacks and water, and that include places to exercise like a gym or walking trail. If you are out of town, try to walk as much as possible instead of being quick to jump into the rental car or hop on public transportation.

59. Spice Up Your Food

Adding a little spice to your food, namely chili peppers, may help with weight loss. There has been some promising research showing that capsaicin, a compound found in chili peppers, may help a bit with metabolism, insulin sensitivity, and weight loss. The evidence is very preliminary, but regardless of its metabolic effects, spicing up your food can add flavor without calories, which helps it to be more palatable and satisfying.

Tips to Make the Habit Stick

- Add chili peppers to dishes like stir-fries and salsas.
- Sprinkle chili pepper on fresh fruit for a sweet and spicy treat.
- Don't like spicy? There are plenty of other great flavors that are not spicy, like ginger, garlic, basil, thyme, and rosemary, to name a few. You can add flavor to your food with spices and herbs to increase palatability without upping calories!

60. Choose a Smaller Plate or Bowl for Eating

Using a smaller plate or bowl to eat foods is an easy way to practice portion control, which in turn will really help your weight and blood sugars. Choose the right-sized plate or bowl for positive portion control.

Tips to Make the Habit Stick

- Use a smaller plate or bowl that won't let you over-portion. It plays a helpful trick by changing your perception that you are eating more. Conversely, avoid using too large of a plate or bowl; that encourages you to take too much or may make your perfectly portioned food look a bit measly.

- To take it one step further, there are now popular portion plates that have sections for you to easily preportion your starch, protein, and veggies without having to weigh and measure.

Chapter 7

Stress Less, Sleep More, and Love More for Your Life

BY NOW YOU know that eating right, exercising, and practicing behavior modification are important steps to managing your prediabetes and improving your overall health. There are some additional factors to consider when dealing with your diagnosis and formulating a successful treatment plan that addresses your whole person. Managing stress and mood, getting adequate rest and good quality sleep, and spending/enjoying time with others can also be very powerful and helpful, as well as have a positive impact on your blood sugar control, weight, and overall health.

Being diagnosed with prediabetes can have a significant emotional impact not just on you but on everyone who lives with and cares for you. Taking good care of yourself and dealing with emotions, learning good coping techniques, and involving others in your journey will help you and those around you live a better, happier life.

Managing Stress: Why Is It So Important?

Experiencing stress doesn't feel good, and it can take a toll on both your mind and body. There are two types of stress: physical and mental. Physical stress occurs when significant demands are placed on the body, such as coping with illness, physical activity that is too intense, or recovering from surgery. Physical stress can have the potential to increase blood sugars and tax other body systems such as the heart. Mental stress originates in our mind—excessive worrying, for example. It also has the potential to wreak havoc on our body's systems, especially if it is chronic, repeated, and long term.

When you face a physically or psychologically stressful situation, your body starts a complex process of hormone release and reaction. The adrenal glands begin to pump out cortisol, the hormone primarily responsible for our physiological "fight-or-flight" reaction to situations we perceive as dangerous. Cortisol signals the liver to start up glucose production to give the brain and central nervous system added energy, while signaling the fat and muscle tissues to slow their uptake. At the same time, it causes the release of fatty acids from fat tissues, which are needed for muscle fuel, and sends your blood pressure up. Stress also prompts the adrenal glands to release epinephrine, the hormone that provides the adrenaline rush of the "fight-or-flight" reaction. High levels of circulating cortisol and epinephrine promote insulin resistance, in addition to ratcheting up blood sugar levels.

Since it increases blood pressure and glucose levels, stress is obviously no good for prediabetes and your health as a whole. In addition to impacting the body and blood sugars directly, stress can also be problematic indirectly because it may distract you from taking proper care of yourself. This is dangerous because it may take you off track from controlling your prediabetes as you become preoccupied with other issues. It can also lead to unhealthy coping mechanisms such as overeating or drinking alcohol.

Does Stress Cause Diabetes?

There is some evidence that extreme, chronic stress may actually cause or predispose an individual to type 2 diabetes. However, stress has also been associated with abdominal or visceral adiposity (that "apple" shape we talked about earlier), so it's unclear whether stress causes a spare tire, and the spare tire causes type 2, or if the link is a more direct one.

Recognizing Stress and Learning to Cope

Let's face it: stress will always be present in our lives one way or another. Whether it's short-term minor woes such as being stuck in traffic or losing your keys, or something larger and long term like tensions in relationships or problems at work, you need to come to terms with your stressors and find healthy ways to cope. Everybody reacts differently to stress, so coping mechanisms may come easier to some and be more difficult for others. Recognizing and becoming aware of when you are stressed is one of the first things you can do to help yourself. Here are some of the signs and symptoms that manifest themselves in our body as reactions to stress:

- **Physical:** fatigue, insomnia, muscle aches, heart palpitations, flushing/sweating, digestive disturbances/abdominal upset, headaches, increased or decreased appetite, frequent cold/illnesses, dry mouth
- **Mental:** anxiety/racing thoughts, difficulty concentrating, nervousness, feeling worried/scared/frustrated/sad/short-tempered/irritable, memory loss

Common negative behavioral reactions to stress include overeating, consuming alcohol or using drugs, becoming withdrawn, having emotional outbursts, pacing, and developing nervous habits like nail-biting. Once you are able to recognize when you are stressed, it is important to find healthy ways to deal with it.

Taking Action and Learning to Cope

Studies have shown that stress-management programs can be extremely effective in improving psychological well-being and blood sugar control. One Duke University study published in *Diabetes Care* found that just five sessions of stress-management training lowered HbA1c levels an average of half a percentage point. The Duke study involved a stress-training regimen of audiotape-led progressive muscle relaxation, cognitive and behavioral therapy (including guided imagery and deep-breathing exercises), and education on the mechanisms and health consequences of stress.

In addition to the guided relaxation, behavioral education, and therapy suggested in this trial, other helpful stress-management techniques include meditation, yoga, music or art therapy, and journaling. Anything that calms you and allows you to relax and release is a good stress-management strategy. Tell someone. Instead of keeping it inside and trying to deal with it on your own, reaching out to your family, friends, and colleagues to talk about a problem can help lessen the burden. And don't forget to seek the help of your medical team and a qualified therapist if you are overwhelmed and having difficulty coping.

The Dangers of Denial

Many people choose to simply ignore that they have prediabetes, continuing as if it didn't exist. The problem with this (non) coping approach is the long-term consequences of uncontrolled blood glucose and weight. By the time they do come to terms with denial and are ready to treat their prediabetes, serious complications may be on their way. Some newly diagnosed patients will acknowledge their feelings of denial. Recognition is a good sign that in the back of your mind you know you must move forward. As long as you're willing to follow your doctor's orders for the time being, even if you haven't fully accepted the condition, denial is a normal part of the process.

Reaching acceptance can be a difficult, rocky road. Many people need the help of a therapist or counselor to get there. A health psychologist who has specialized training in the intricate psychological, biological, and social relationships between physical illness and mental health can be helpful in sorting through coping issues.

Feeling Guilty

It may not be rational, but it's perfectly normal to feel guilty about having prediabetes. But now that you know it's normal, it's time to move on. You are not entirely to blame for having prediabetes, nor should you feel ashamed of your diagnosis. Realize that your genetic makeup and/ or environmental factors may have made you susceptible to it and try to view it as a positive wake-up call to improve certain lifestyle habits and behaviors, like beginning a healthy diet and starting regular exercise, as a way to make lifelong changes for the better.

A Word about Depression

Up to 30 percent of people with diabetes also suffer from symptoms of depression, and people with diabetes are twice as likely to become clinically depressed than are those without diabetes. Some studies have also seen a moderate increase in the prevalence of depression in those with prediabetes. Occasional sadness, fear, and uncertainty are normal in prediabetes, but when they start affecting your everyday enjoyment of life and interfering with proper self-care, they may be something more than just a passing emotional downturn. Depression can be treated with therapy and/or antidepressant medication, so there's no reason to suffer needlessly. Here are a few other points that may help you deal with depression:

- *Knowledge is power.* Fear of the unknown can feed your depression. If you haven't already done so, start educating yourself about your condition.
- *Seek support.* Draw on the experience and emotional comfort of your family, friends, spiritual community, healthcare team, and others with prediabetes/diabetes.
- *Keep perfection in perspective.* Reward your successes, big or small, and try to see your stumbles as learning experiences rather than failures.
- *Don't stop moving.* Push yourself to take a brisk walk daily. Exercise raises your level of endorphins and is a natural mood booster.

Know the Signs of Depression

Common signs of a depressive disorder include weight loss, insomnia (too little sleep) or hypersomnia (too much sleep), irritability or agitation, fatigue, feelings of guilt or worthlessness, inability to concentrate, and recurrent thoughts of death or suicide.

Sleep: Why Is It So Important?

The importance of a good night's sleep should never be underestimated. It can make all the difference to your physical and mental health. Adequate sleep quality and quantity are essential to maintaining several key processes in the body such as release of hormones, regulation of metabolism, controlling appetite and weight, and upkeep of proper immune system and brain function. It is no wonder that sleep deprivation has been linked to a multitude of problems such as:

- Increased risk of diseases like cardiovascular disease, kidney disease, obesity
- Susceptibility to infections, like the common cold
- Emotional and behavioral problems, like increased stress, lower cognitive function (reduced ability to learn and concentrate), and depression
- Lack of safety, such as more accidents and errors and issues with judgment

In addition, many studies have found that poor sleep quality and inadequate quantity may be linked to prediabetes, diabetes, and metabolic syndrome. Sleep plays a major role in helping the endocrine system function, namely the regulation of glucose metabolism. Poor sleep can lead to insulin resistance. The sleep-waking cycle and length of sleeping time have a lot to do with helping control glucose tolerance and insulin secretion. Inadequate sleep can also change levels of hormones that regulate appetite, which leads to excessive food consumption, resulting in obesity.

How Much Sleep Do You Really Need?

The amount of sleep your body requires varies with age. According to the National Sleep Foundation's (NSF) expert panel, the following are the recommended amounts of sleep per night for various age groups across the life span:

- Newborns (0–3 months): 14–17 hours
- Infants (4–11 months): 12–15 hours
- Toddlers (1–2 years): 11–13 hours
- Preschoolers (3–5 years): 10–13 hours
- School-age children (6–13 years): 9–11 hours
- Teenagers (14–17 years): 8–10 hours
- Young adults/adults (18–25 years/26–64 years): 7–8 hours
- Older adults (65 years or older): 7–8 hours

What about Sleep Quality?

It's not just the quantity of sleep you get that's important; the quality of your sleep also matters. The latest report by the NSF in 2017 listed the key indicators of good quality sleep as the following:

- Sleeping most of the time while in bed (at least 85 percent of total time)
- Falling asleep in thirty minutes or less
- Waking up no more than once per night
- Being awake for twenty minutes or less after initially falling asleep

Why Are We Not Getting Enough Sleep?

There have been quite a few changes in human sleep habits over the past several decades; some studies and surveys suggest we are potentially sleeping fewer hours than we used to. The modern lifestyle that is characterized by obsession with electronic devices, longer work hours, night-shift work, and longer waking hours of days packed with activities poses a huge challenge to getting adequate sleep.

Lacking in the Sleep Department

According to a recent study in the CDC's *Morbidity and Mortality Weekly Report*, more than one-third of adult Americans are not getting adequate sleep on a regular basis.

The reality is that for many of us, getting enough sleep is just not a priority. However, the potential for good rest is there if we take advantage of it. Yet for some, sleep disorders create challenges to falling asleep and getting good quality sleep.

What Is Obstructive Sleep Apnea?

Obstructive sleep apnea (OSA) is a common sleep disorder that occurs in approximately 3–7 percent of the general population. Individuals with OSA experience blockages in the airway repeatedly during sleep, sometimes blocking breathing entirely. Common causes include a person's physical structure, such as large tonsils or medical conditions like obesity and neuromuscular disorders. OSA may lead to impaired glucose tolerance and/or insulin sensitivity, so there is a higher prevalence of the condition among those with prediabetes and diabetes. There are other complications in people with OSA. The condition is diagnosed by a sleep study and is most often treated by the use of breathing devices as well as lifestyle changes.

Insomnia

As many as 10 percent of adults in the US experience chronic insomnia, a common sleep disorder that is characterized by difficulty falling asleep, staying asleep, waking up too early, and not feeling well rested. There are many causes of insomnia ranging from medical issues and medication side effects to mental health problems such as stress and anxiety. Researchers also factor in aging; gender (women are more prone to insomnia than men); use of stimulants such as caffeine, alcohol, or nicotine; or changes in schedule due to work shifts and traveling.

If you are having trouble with chronic insomnia, it is important to discuss it with your medical team so you can work together to try to find the causes and create a treatment plan. Example treatments for insomnia are lifestyle changes, behavioral therapy, medications, and relaxation techniques. If you think you may have insomnia or other sleep problems, don't hesitate to seek help from a medical professional. Also, review some of the healthy habits later in this chapter for some simple tips and changes that may make a difference so you can get enough quality sleep, something that is an integral part of managing your prediabetes.

Social Support: A Positive Factor

Maintaining a social support network is good for your health and is a key component to helping you deal with your prediabetes diagnosis and manage it successfully. Countless studies have shown that having social support from others can have direct effects on health, such as improving blood sugar control, helping with weight management, and lowering stress and depression.

Social support can take on many forms, all of which can be beneficial in different ways. The types of social support that can help with managing prediabetes include:

- **Emotional support:** affection, love, care, empathy, trust building
- **Esteem support:** encouragement of independence and reinforcement of self-care and skills/abilities
- **Informational support:** recommendations, facts, advice, information
- **Tangible support:** help with tasks from others, financial assistance
- **Social network support:** sense of belonging to a group, companionship and identification

As you can see, there are many, many ways you can get support from others, so try to take advantage of their benefits. Reach out to those you are close to and feel comfortable with. Your support network can and should include your family, friends, work colleagues, peers with your medical condition, and your healthcare team. Check Appendix C at the end of this book for some online support group examples and suggestions.

Help Them Help You

This section is good to share with those who support you. In order to get the benefits of social support, you need to be able to accept help from others. Some people may offer it automatically, and other times you will need to ask and make your needs known.

Information for Spouses, Loved Ones, and Family Members

When your partner or family member is handed a prediabetes diagnosis, so are you. Get onboard with a management plan right off the bat. You can and should educate yourself and read this book to learn more about the condition and how to treat it. If you do the grocery shopping and/or cooking in your household, you should absolutely attend the meeting your partner/family member has with a registered dietitian. And if your partner feels comfortable with it, go along on doctor's visits as well. Two sets of ears are always better than one.

Try (and it can be hard) not to become the prediabetes patrol. Think of what it would be like to go through life listening to the following:

- "Are you sure you can eat that?"
- "Do you really think you should have that?"
- "Don't you think you should do something about that blood sugar reading?"

Communicate openly and honestly with your partner or family member about how you can help when things aren't going right, before they go astray. That way you know in advance what is the most effective way to assist.

Helping Those Who Don't Help Themselves

Perhaps you're reading this book because you're more interested in prediabetes control than your family member or significant other—the one with the condition—is. Maybe they haven't come to terms with their diagnosis yet, or maybe they are depressed or disheartened and have stopped trying. You can read and learn until you're blue in the face, and you may even be able to nag your family member or partner into exercising here or there or eating a more appropriate meal. But you can't control their diabetes for them. Remember this if you remember nothing else: your mental health and emotional well-being are just as important as theirs, and you can save yourself countless hours of head-banging frustration if you detach enough to realize that they are the captain of the prediabetes ship.

Don't Overstep Boundaries

Support your family member or partner, but keep in mind that they, and not you, are in charge of taking care of their prediabetes. This means being there for them if they ask you for help, offering to go to the doctor's appointments—but not pushing the issue—and not eating things right in front of them that they can't have.

At the same time, you don't want to go too far in the other direction and make it easier for your family member or partner to get away with screwing up their control by going along with their program. Accepting the excuses about why that extra piece of pie just had to be eaten or nodding your head when they say, "I'm going to exercise tomorrow" is not being supportive. It's called "enabling," and spouses and family members of alcoholics do it all the time. Don't let yourself become part of the problem or validate bad behaviors.

Caring for Children with Prediabetes

Prediabetes affects the entire family—beyond the lifestyle adjustments a family is faced with, there is fear, guilt, jealousy, anger, and other emotions to come to terms with. Both the parent-child and the sibling relationships can face difficult challenges that require empathy, discipline, and flexibility to work through and beyond.

Whether it is a parent or child who has prediabetes, the whole family can benefit from diabetes education classes. Even small children can learn more about the disease through age-appropriate books. It's easy to feel isolated when you have prediabetes, and involvement of the family goes a long way toward creating a caring and supportive environment that makes control easier.

To Love and Not Overprotect

If your child has prediabetes, he or she has more boundaries than others, and it can be easy to fall into the trap of making them tighter than necessary. Letting your fears overtake your child's normal social development is not healthy for either of you. Kids need to be kids—to participate in sports, to go to birthday parties, to spend the day at the beach with friends, and to go to school dances and football games. Follow the "first do no harm" motto of the medical profession and take the least-invasive route when making decisions about what your child can and cannot do, based on your child's age, responsibility, and level of competence with her or his own prediabetes care. If you must say no, let your child know the reasoning behind the decision. "Because I said so" is not a good explanation and will not help to make boundaries clearer to your son or daughter.

As your child grows and takes a greater deal of control over her own care, you may find yourself feeling strangely unneeded. Remember that your adolescent is forming her own identity and needs the autonomy to make some of her own treatment decisions and take over more of her day-to-day management. You do need to remain a partner in her care, however.

Caregivers Need Care, Too

While it gets easier with practice and age, it's emotionally exhausting to stand guard over your child day in and day out. Arrange for backup care for your child at least once a month and get out and enjoy yourself. You might also check out the availability of support groups for parents of children with health conditions in your area as both a sounding board and shoulder to lean on.

Support Groups: We're in This Together

Support groups are an absolutely invaluable resource for adults with prediabetes, diabetes, and weight issues. A support group offers patients a chance to compare treatment notes, to talk about emotional issues in living with health issues, and to air their gripes about the healthcare system.

In addition to expanding your knowledge and fostering a sense of cama-raderie, a support group is a good stress-release valve.

Your doctor's office and/or local hospital are good places to check on existing support groups. If you find that your community doesn't have one, ask your physician, dietitian, or behavior therapist about the possible interest level in a group among other patients. You may be able to set up one of your own. There are also many online support groups available for diabetes and a variety of health conditions.

The Power of Love?

Can a healthy dose of love be an actual treatment for predia-betes? The answer is quite possibly. Recent studies have revealed that oxytocin, often referred to as a "love hormone," may improve health in prediabetes, diabetes, and metabolic syndrome by low-ering insulin resistance, improving glucose tolerance, and weight loss. Levels of oxytocin increase in the body after positive phys-ical contact such as hugging, massage, sexual intercourse, and breastfeeding. More research is underway to investigate uses of synthetic oxytocin and its potential to help health conditions, but for now human contact with loved ones is the best and most nat-ural source.

Now let's turn to habits that will help you stress less, sleep more, and love more! All of these are important building blocks in the project of managing and reversing your prediabetes.

61. Harness the Power of Deep Breathing

If you find that you are feeling stressed, foggy, anxious, or upset, one of the best things you can do is to take time out and breathe. The simple act of just taking a few deep breaths can help calm your body and clear your mind, not to mention that it can do wonders for your blood sugars. Focus on simple breathing to help relax and use it as a simple, healthy coping mechanism.

Tips to Make the Habit Stick

- A simple breathing technique is to sit in a chair, close your eyes, and take a deep, slow breath. Hold it in for a few seconds and then breath out fully and very slowly for a few seconds. Repeat this up to five to ten times to help relax and reset.
- Instead of succumbing to unhealthy coping mechanisms like junk food, alcohol, or tuning out and withdrawing, take time out to acknowledge the way you are feeling and give yourself a moment to breathe.

62. Consider Meditation

Quite a few studies have shown that meditation is very beneficial to health. Primarily, it reduces stress. It has been demonstrated that meditation can have positive effects on multiple areas in the body, including our metabolic, endocrine, and psychological systems. It can even lower insulin resistance, blood sugar, and hemoglobin A1c. Consider meditation to help clear your mind and relax your body for stress reduction.

Tips to Make the Habit Stick

- For guidance and instruction, try taking a meditation class. You can also use a meditation DVD or app in the comfort of your own home.
- Try programs that combine meditation with yoga so you can get the added benefit of stretching and strengthening, which counts as physical activity too.
- Practice and don't give up. Meditation takes time to learn and requires intense focus on breathing and mental concentration, but the effort will be worth it.

63. Practice Healthy Coping

If you find yourself becoming stressed, know that it is not good for your prediabetes. Make sure to take time out for yourself to give your mind and body a break. Take your mind off the stress and give yourself time to relax. When you give yourself some time out, you can reapproach your problem with a clearer mind.

Tips to Make the Habit Stick

- Engage in positive activities to cope such as:
  - Exercising, even taking a simple walk
  - Doing a hobby you enjoy, such as playing sports, crafting, or dancing
  - Reading a good book
  - Spending time with friends and family
  - Going out to see a movie
  - Taking a warm bath
  - Meditating or doing some deep breathing
  - Writing it down—journaling your thoughts

64. Don't Go It Alone

If you are experiencing stress and worry, don't keep it inside and try to deal with it entirely by yourself. Lean on others in your support system in times of stress; it can make a big difference.

Tips to Make the Habit Stick

- Reach out for help by talking about your feelings with family, friends, or a colleague to vent and take advantage of companionship.
- Consider seeing a behavioral therapist for persistent stress and mood changes such as depression or anxiety to discuss your issues and learn ways to cope.
- Think about joining a support group to interact with others who can identify with what you are going through. You might be surprised how relieved you feel after letting out what is bothering you, and it can certainly help you manage your prediabetes as well.

65. Reframe Your Thoughts

If you find that negative or worrisome thoughts are bringing you down, try to replace them or put a positive spin on your thoughts instead. Use the power of positive thinking to help you through difficult times.

Tips to Make the Habit Stick

- Make attempts to see the best in situations as often as you can. For example, if you are thinking, "I dread doing this project; it's so much work, and it's going to be terrible," instead try, "Wow, this project is going to be challenging, but I can do it. I will take it a step at a time, and it will feel awesome when I get it done."
- Sometimes it's helpful to have a mantra or upbeat saying that you can repeat to yourself over and over. Combining it with deep breathing can combat mental stress, which is key to blood sugar control.

66. Laugh and Smile More

Never underestimate the power of a good hearty laugh. Did you know that scientific studies have demonstrated the health benefits of laughter? These include helping cardiovascular functions and delaying complications in type 2 diabetes. It's true. Laughter causes positive changes that affect us for the better psychologically, biochemically, and in terms of our immunity. So go ahead, laugh and smile more. Lighten up. Your body and mind will thank you for it!

Tips to Make the Habit Stick

- Read a funny story, the comics, or watch a comedy show or movie.
- Tell jokes and funny stories around the table for some planned silliness with your family and friends.

67. Help Yourself by Helping Others

If you are feeling down, stressed, or in a rut, consider volunteering. Preliminary studies have shown that volunteering can lower depression and mortality and can increase feelings of well-being. Consider reaching out to others to help them, and you may just help yourself in the process.

Tips to Make the Habit Stick

- Find a cause that you are interested in or passionate about such as helping animals, the elderly, or the less fortunate. Helping others can help you be more social, create a sense of purpose, and just make you feel good.

- Make sure you have a healthy life balance with volunteer work so it doesn't become too much for your schedule and actually cause stress. Decide on a regular time commitment that works best for you to help out.

- Volunteering doesn't always have to be done through a formal organization; sometimes just taking time to help a family member, a friend, or a neighbor with a project or an errand can be a way of lending a hand.

68. Create an Environment Conducive to Sleep

Check your room to determine if it is sleep-friendly. Do your best to create a comfortable bedroom that encourages sleep and helps you to promote control of your prediabetes and health.

Tips to Make the Habit Stick

- Make sure your bed is large enough and your pillow is comfortable. A good mattress can be helpful and should not be older than nine or ten years.

- Your room should be as dark and as quiet as possible. If it is not, then consider using a sleep blindfold, earplugs, or blackout curtains.

- You will also want to keep the room well ventilated and at the right temperature as well, not too hot or too cold for you.

69. Try to Stick to a Regular Sleep Schedule

By keeping a habitual bedtime and waking time you can help set your body's internal clock, referred to as a circadian rhythm, in your favor. This will help to get you adapted to a good sleep routine. Also, by keeping to a regular bedtime your schedule can help ensure you will get to bed in time to get enough hours of sleep. Create a sleep schedule for more consistent rest as an important part of your prediabetes management.

Tips to Make the Habit Stick

- Make every attempt to go to bed around the same time every night, even on the weekends, if possible. Try not to sleep in more than one or two hours maximum on the weekends or days off. Large shifts in your bedtime or waking hours can disrupt your circadian rhythm and cause problems with sleep as well as your alertness and energy levels during the day.

- If you are trying to adjust to an earlier bedtime, do it gradually in fifteen-minute intervals each night until the routine is comfortable.

- Have trouble waking up in the morning? Let some morning sunlight in to help your internal body clock work with you to greet the day.

70. Develop a Calming Bedtime Ritual

Give yourself some time to wind down the hour before bed—your body and blood sugars will thank you for it. Do your best to relax before bedtime in as many ways as possible.

Tips to Make the Habit Stick

- Avoid bright lights up to an hour before bedtime and keep things as dim as possible to prevent disrupting your internal clock and to encourage sleepiness.
- As difficult as it may be, skip computers, TV, tablets, and cell phones up to an hour before turning in. The blue light they emit may be disruptive and keep you from falling asleep.
- Instead of using electronics, do some light reading, listen to music, talk with a loved one about your day, or even take a warm bath or shower to help relax your body and get ready for bed.

71. Avoid Sleep Saboteurs

There are some things to watch out for near bedtime that can prevent a good night's sleep. And remember that a sound sleep helps to control your prediabetes. Don't engage in behaviors that prevent sleep.

Tips to Make the Habit Stick

- Avoid caffeine—cut the coffee, tea, and cola before bed since they are stimulants. If you must drink coffee, switch to decaf, but be aware it still has some caffeine. Watch foods and beverages containing chocolate or too much sugar as well.
- Don't consume too little or too much food close to bedtime. Being hungry before bed can make it difficult to fall asleep, but feeling stuffed can be uncomfortable and cause indigestion that may keep you awake.
- Be careful about late afternoon naps—too much napping can disrupt your body's internal clock and make it difficult to get to sleep on time.

72. If Trouble Sleeping Is a Chronic Problem, Get Help

Have you tried everything and are still having trouble getting to sleep or staying asleep? In that case it may be time to see the doctor to investigate the causes and work on a treatment plan together. Reach out to professionals for guidance for persistent sleep troubles.

Tips to Make the Habit Stick

- If psychological issues such as stress, anxiety, or depression are troubling you, then seeing a doctor and behavioral therapist can help you tackle these barriers that may be preventing your sleep. Remember that a good night's sleep every night is key to your prediabetes management plan.
- Keep notes or a journal of your sleep and mood as this can be helpful to bring to appointments and can increase your awareness of barriers that may be preventing sleep.

73. Use Regular Exercise As a Natural Sleep Aide

By now you have read about all the benefits of exercise—it helps improve blood sugar control and weight. Well, it can also help you sleep!

Tips to Make the Habit Stick

- Keep active daily to take advantage of all the positive effects of exercise, including better sleep. Conversely, improved sleep can help motivate you to do regular activity.
- Use regular exercise to promote body changes that promote sleep. It can help reduce stress, depression, and anxiety, and it may promote changes in body temperature and circadian rhythms, all of which can encourage sleep.

74. Help Others Help You

If you are lucky enough to have people around you offering love and support, embrace it and tell them how they can help. Take advantage of your support by giving others some direction about how to help.

Tips to Make the Habit Stick

- Use clear communication so your friends and family can get on the same page about what your needs are and how they can best assist and support you during your prediabetes treatment.
- Be open and specific to eliminate any confusion or hesitation they may have as to how they can help. Give them examples of how to help. This can turn their good intentions into concrete actions that will benefit you and your relationship. In turn, this can improve your health and adherence to your treatment plan.

75. Do Date Nights

With our busy lifestyles it is easy to get caught up in the monotony of our jobs and other commitments, which can take too much time away from relationships with your partner, family, and friends. Carving out regular time is important to maintaining love and social connections that strengthen bonds and maintain the support network that is so beneficial to your mental and physical health. Taking this time can help you succeed in managing your prediabetes. Schedule time to connect with your loved ones to promote healthy relationships and, in turn, a healthy body and mind.

Tips to Make the Habit Stick

- Plan a regular date night with your partner to take time out to connect and have fun without distractions.
- Schedule outings with your family so you can spend quality time together to talk, laugh, and enjoy each other's company.
- Spend a night out with friends, catching up and reminiscing.

76. Consider Counseling

If constant clashes are creating tension and stress between you and your partner or with other members of your family, then consider going to counseling together. Get some guidance on how to create stronger and healthier relationships so tension will not take a toll on your blood sugar and body.

Tips to Make the Habit Stick

- Look for a therapist who specializes in marriage and family therapy. Going together can be a way to spend time working on problems where you are all engaged and involved.
- Don't wait too long to get help. Remember, stress can take a toll on your blood sugar, weight, and health, so getting to the root of your problems and working things out sooner than later will benefit your health as well as those around you.

77. Acknowledge Intimacy Issues

Regular intimacy and sex can be very good for your health and the health of your relationship, so it's best to try to tackle any barriers that are getting in the way.

If you are having problems in the bedroom, it is okay to talk about it and get some help.

Tips to Make the Habit Stick

- If you are having trouble connecting with your partner intimately, be open with her or him about it and discuss the possibility of seeking professional help. Eliminating intimacy issues with your partner can decrease the stress and tension that take a toll on your health and blood sugars. Dealing with these issues also opens the door to the beneficial effects that physical connections can have on your mind and body. Be honest about problems with intimacy with your partner and work on ways to reconnect and enjoy life together.

- If your prediabetes is causing changes in your body that are making sex uncomfortable, or if stress and mood changes are interfering with your sex drive, then seek out guidance from your doctor and possibly a therapist.

- Carve out some time to connect with your partner physically and mentally each day. Plan date nights or weekend getaways to keep your relationship fun, romantic, and interesting.

78. Learn More about Prediabetes and Its Treatment Together

The diagnosis of prediabetes can be overwhelming and emotional. Let your partner, family, and friends take the journey with you by learning more about the condition and the lifestyle changes that are required.

Tips to Make the Habit Stick

- Having your partner and/or family members at medical appointments can be helpful. It's good to have more than one set of ears in case you have trouble remembering or understanding recommendations. If you and your friends and family are all clear on the condition and its treatment plan, you'll be more effective in managing your prediabetes.
- Let others go with you to your appointment with the dietitian, especially if your partner does the cooking or the grocery shopping. That way she or he can support your meal plan.
- Remind yourself that it can be a positive experience to have others on your team as you are starting to get familiar with prediabetes and how to tackle it.

79. Use Your Online Resources

How many times have we heard that there is a wealth of information on just about any subject on the Internet? This is also the case for prediabetes and diabetes. Using online information and support can be helpful as resources to enhance your prediabetes treatment plan. If you have a question, get in the habit of looking up the answer.

Tips to Make the Habit Stick

- Take advantage of the Internet to get more information about your condition and for helpful lifestyle change ideas—especially recipes and menu ideas.

- Make sure your sources are reputable, as there is a lot of misinformation online too. Consult the list of resources in Appendix C at the end of this book.

- Investigate online support communities. There are many online groups for people with prediabetes, diabetes, and obesity, and they can be almost as—if not more—supportive and informative than real-time groups. There's input from Pennsylvania to Paris, with participants from all walks of life and a broad range of experience with these health conditions. On the other hand, you may get inaccurate medical information from people who either don't know better or who are trying to sell some miracle cure, so beware of accepting specific medical advice from random people online and always run new ideas by your doctor. The "miracle" workers can be taken care of by the moderator, using a firm hand. As long as you take what you read with a grain of salt, you certainly stand more to gain than you can lose. The beauty of an online support group is that it is there all day and all night for your questions, vents, and gripes.

80. Make Lifestyle Change a Family Affair

If you have been diagnosed with prediabetes, or if a family member has, then make needed changes in diet, exercise, and behavior together. Everyone in the household can benefit from eating a healthy diet, getting more activity, getting more sleep, and engaging in positive behavior for health. The family that sticks to important lifestyle changes stays healthy together!

Tips to Make the Habit Stick

- Get everyone onboard with your plan so there is less temptation to eat the wrong things or slack off on activity. You can all help motivate each other.
- Do healthy activities together like going shopping and cooking a nutritious meal together, doing group exercise sessions like biking or hiking, and taking time out to relax as a family with upbeat activities like a family game night or a dance party. These are just a few of many ways to spend quality time to bond together as a family and strengthen your relationships.

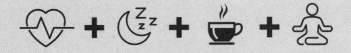

Chapter 8

Develop Problem-Solving Habits for Your Life

DIABETES AND PREDIABETES can be complex and challenging to manage, and a large part of their treatment is about making lifestyle changes. You need a comprehensive plan to address a variety of issues in order to make the right choices and develop healthy habits. One of the keys to success in making changes and maintaining them is having good problem-solving abilities.

Problem-Solving: One of the Key Components of Self-Care

It has been well documented that problem-solving is a core skill to have for effective prediabetes and diabetes self-management. This is so much the case that certified diabetes educators are urged to focus on problem-solving in the AADE7 Self-Care Behaviors outlined by the American Association of Diabetes Educators (AADE). This is a framework of seven self-care behaviors that are an effective way to make positive changes in lifestyle. Take a look at these behaviors; most of them also apply to those with prediabetes:

The Seven Self-Care Behaviors

1. **Healthy Eating:** Make healthy food choices, understand portion sizes, and learn the best times to eat.

2. **Being Active:** Include regular activity for overall fitness, weight management, and blood glucose control.

3. **Monitoring:** Daily self-monitor blood glucose to assess how food, physical activity, and medications are working.

4. **Taking Medication:** Understand how medications work and when to take them.

5. **Problem-Solving:** Know how to problem solve. For example, a high or low blood glucose episode could require you to make a quick decision about food, activity, or medication.

6. **Reducing Risks:** Effective risk-reduction behaviors such as smoking cessation and regular eye exams are examples of self-care that reduce risk of complications.

7. **Healthy Coping:** Good coping skills that deal with the challenges of diabetes help people stay motivated to keep their diabetes in control.

What Is a Certified Diabetes Educator?

A Certified Diabetes Educator (CDE) is a health professional who has in-depth knowledge and experience in diabetes prevention, prediabetes, and diabetes management. Many are registered dietitians, nurses, or pharmacists who have chosen to get additional education and certification to work more closely in the area of diabetes.

This book has addressed and given many tips for most of these behaviors for self-care, but let's explore problem-solving in a bit more detail.

The Logistics of Problem-Solving

According to the AADE principles, problem-solving is a continuous cycle of four main steps: (1) Act (2) Analyze and Evaluate (3) Discuss Solutions (4) Learn from Experience (then repeat!). Problem-solving is a learned behavior of identifying a problem, selecting and applying the best strategy to solve it, and evaluating the effectiveness of that strategy choice. By figuring out the barriers to your self-care and then tackling them, you can be more successful in making the needed lifestyle changes such as eating a good diet, engaging in regular activity, losing weight, and other changes you should make to treat your prediabetes.

Everyone has different attitudes and approaches to problem-solving. Some are more successful, skilled, and positive than others. A problem may be viewed as a challenge by some but may also be seen as a threat by others. In addition to your attitude about the issue and the skills you possess to approach a problem, factors such as past experience with the problem and knowledge about the disease or condition can also determine how successful you are in dealing with prediabetes and diabetes-related issues.

Approaching a Problem

When faced with a problem, it is important to be honest with yourself about what is happening. You need to try to understand why the problem has arisen and to learn from it—all of which will probably help you in the future. Keep in mind these tips:

- **Admit you have a problem:** Don't ignore it or be too hard on yourself; everyone faces problems throughout life.
- **Pause and analyze why the problem is occurring:** What is different with you and your routine this time around?
- **Correct and learn from the problem:** Try to solve it in the way that you think makes sense…brainstorm about the possibilities. Often you can look back to how you successfully dealt with similar problems in the past.
- **Get help with your problem:** Evaluate your solutions and improve upon them with the guidance of family, friends, and, if needed, your doctor or therapist.
- **Test out new solutions:** Problem-solving can often be a process of trial and error; find what works best for you and stick with those strategies.

No matter how much you plan to achieve your goals and manage prediabetes, unexpected problems can come up that you will need to face and deal with. Remember that prediabetes self-care starts with *you* and that the day-to-day management of your condition is in your hands. The victory is yours if you want it. By obtaining the right amount of knowledge about the condition, practicing problem-solving skills, taking advantage of your support systems, and keeping a positive attitude, *you* have the power to be successful in making changes to improve your lifestyle habits, to conquer prediabetes, and to have a happier and healthier life.

Here are some problem-solving habits that will help you manage and reverse your prediabetes.

81. *Don't* Skip Meals and Fluids, *Do* Set Regular Times for Meals, Snacks, and Hydration

Even if you are busy, that is no excuse to skimp on meals and miss out on enough fluid intake. Missing a meal or snack can zap your energy, lead to headaches and irritability, and set you up for making poor food choices. Skipping regular meals often leads you to eat excess portions once you do allow yourself to eat. This can cause trouble with your blood sugars and weight. Losing out on drinking water can lead to dehydration and dry mouth. Factor in your ways to fuel and hydrate ahead of time to get into a good routine and avoid missing out on needed food and fluids.

Tips to Make the Habit Stick

- Make sure to plan ahead each day when and where your meals are going to be. Keep water with you at all times. Prepare meals and snacks to have ready at home or to take with you at school, work, or on the go.

- Know ahead of time if you are going to be eating out so you can develop a strategy to make reasonable food choices.

- Drink a glass of water before and after meals. Keep a large reusable water container with you at your desk, on the go, or at your bedside.

- Set an alarm or timer to remind you to eat or drink.

82. *Don't* Sabotage Yourself When Eating Out, *Do* Control Your Portions and Choices

Many people consider restaurant meals a special occasion, and this can mean a time to splurge on desserts or rich foods. If you dine out too often, viewing all meals out as special occasions will undermine your efforts to eat healthier and control your prediabetes. Be smart in your food choices when eating out and only splurge occasionally in a way that is planned.

Tips to Make the Habit Stick

- Take a closer look at how often you dine out, the type of food you order, and how much of this food you eat. This can help you assess what changes you may need to make. Sharing this information with a dietitian can be helpful in identifying patterns that are helping or hindering your progress.

- Take time to figure out healthy food choices at your favorite restaurants that you frequent so you can take the guesswork out of what to order.

- Plan to cheat once in a while by enjoying small portions of foods that you love. Balance this with other lower-calorie choices at meals before and after your cheat meal.

83. *Don't* Fall off the Wagon Because of a Slip-Up, *Do* Move on

If you haven't already, at one point in your life you will probably end up with an "Oh, wow!" or "Yikes!" feeling after splurging on something you shouldn't have. Prediabetes can certainly be a condition of highs and lows, both physically and emotionally. Strive to achieve balance in the emotional area as well as the physical one.

Tips to Make the Habit Stick

- Ask yourself if there was a specific trigger for the slip-up. Maybe you had a particularly stressful day at work or went to a party hungry?
- If you can pinpoint a cause, think about how you can prevent it from happening next time, whether by adjusting your eating schedule or learning some stress-management techniques.
- Don't be too hard on yourself and learn from your mistake. It is not the end of the world if you slip up. If you're too busy kicking yourself for your mistake, you'll miss any lesson you might gain. Be honest with yourself about the mistake, don't sweat it, and regain control.

84. *Don't* Fall Into the Takeout Trap, *Do* Try to Eat More Meals at Home

For many Americans, work schedules and busy lifestyles have made restaurant dining and ordering takeout a common and frequent occurrence. This can present lots of challenges when your goals are to maintain a healthy eating plan, control blood sugars, and lose weight.

Tips to Make the Habit Stick

- Reexamine why you are eating out or ordering food in so much. Maybe you are not making adequate time to eat and are making frequent visits to fast-food restaurants in a rush. Perhaps you're eating out often or frequently getting delivery because you do not keep enough healthy foods available at home.

- If you eat out to be with friends and to be social, try nonfood-related activities in order to spend time together. Go for a walk, meet at a friend's or family member's house to catch up, or go out to a movie.

- To increase the number of meals you prepare and eat at home, take time out each week to make a meal list, grocery shop, and make some healthy meals and snacks in advance to have ready to go when you don't have time to cook. This way you can control your portions, know what ingredients are in your food, and save some money too! Plan ahead to keep healthy foods around at home so you reduce the temptation to eat out.

85. *Don't* Use Food As Your Go-To Reward, *Do* Celebrate Your Successes

Sure, there are many celebrations and holidays that are associated with food: the Fourth of July with hot dogs and hamburgers, Thanksgiving with turkey, and so on. Birthdays and parties can involve a lot of eating and drinking (that will be addressed in the next tip). However, that doesn't mean you need to acknowledge your own successes with food too. Be creative with fun nonfood ways to reward yourself that will not add pounds or increase blood sugars.

Tips to Make the Habit Stick

- Make a list of things you love to do that are nonfood-related and pick one of them when you meet a lifestyle goal. That way you will have a healthy nonfood treat option coming your way as a festive way to reward yourself without adding to your waistline and increasing your blood sugars.
- Plan to see a movie, go shopping for new clothes, try a yoga class, or treat yourself to a massage. These are just a few of many ways that you can treat yourself without food.

86. *Don't* Overindulge When at Gatherings, *Do* Plan Ahead

Go into a gathering with a plan and the right mind-set so you will not come out with extra pounds and higher blood sugars. There are plenty of ways to navigate special occasions without sabotaging your prediabetes treatment plan.

Tips to Make the Habit Stick

- If you are comfortable with having your condition known, let your host know you are prediabetic and inquire about the food offerings so you can figure out your meal in advance.

- Bring a healthy item or two to share to ensure you will have something reasonable to choose from, such as crudités with low-fat dip, a salad, or cut-up fruit/mixed berries.

- When at the event, portion your choices sensibly and move away from the table of food to resist extra servings. Don't eat while standing.

- Help yourself to extra servings of water and other low-calorie beverages to help keep you full without adding calories.

- Make the gathering more about catching up on conversation and less about the food.

- If you are the host, send any treats or excess leftovers home with your guests or bring them into your office or that book club or poker night session coming up so they don't remain at home to tempt you.

87. *Don't* Let Family and Friends Disrupt Your Lifestyle Plan, *Do* Get Them Onboard with Your Goals

Your loved ones need to know what your goals and plans are in terms of your prediabetes treatment so they can be supportive and encourage you to meet them. Work together with those around you, not against each other, when it comes to the upkeep of your prediabetes treatment plan.

Tips to Make the Habit Stick

- As mentioned before, it is best that you and your family are all following a similar lifestyle plan, especially when it comes to eating. However, if that's not the case, ask them not to keep tempting food in the house or indulge themselves when you are together.
- Make your friends and family aware if you feel that they are doing things that are creating barriers to your prediabetes treatment goals. Be honest and have respectful communication.
- Seek the help of your medical team such as a therapist and dietitian if you need more guidance on how to get your family and friends more in tune with your plan and goals.

88. *Don't* Shut Others Out, *Do* Let People In

Realize you do not need to deal with stress and your problems alone. It's okay to spend some healthy alone time here and there, but isolating yourself entirely can only add to your stress and leave you more susceptible to unhealthy coping mechanisms like emotional eating or being inactive. This can sabotage your ability to control your prediabetes. Open up and seek help from therapists, support groups, and family.

Tips to Make the Habit Stick

- Take small steps to share what you feel comfortable with and talk about the most important issues that you need to address first.
- Make a weekly date with family and friends to keep communication lines open and consider regular sessions with a therapist if your troubles become overwhelming.
- Pick up a phone and reach out to someone if you are having a rough moment.

89. *Don't* Put Off Exercise, *Do* It Today and Most Days

If you have a superbusy life and don't set aside a specific time for exercise, then the days will pass you by, and you will miss out. There are no excuses—unless you are ill or have an injury because of which your doctor recommends you abstain from activity. Plan to fill your days with at least thirty minutes total of activity.

Tips to Make the Habit Stick

- Look at your schedule and figure out time slots when you can be active. Your prediabetes control depends on it.
- Multitask and make plans with family and friends that center on exercise. Spend time together being active and staying fit. Walk or bike to work or to do your errands, if it is possible to do so.
- Sign up for an exercise class near your office or home. Don't give yourself even a minute to talk yourself out of it. Just get your workout clothes on, lace up your athletic shoes, and go do it.
- Take a walk at lunch or have your family join you for one after dinner.
- Meet up with your exercise buddy on a weekly basis to be social while you are active.
- Make a list of all the ways you can be active, using tips from Chapter 5. Add them into each of your days and put them on your schedule. Remember that even five or ten minutes of activity a few times a day adds up.

90. *Don't* Get Bored with Your Lifestyle Routine, *Do* Mix It Up

Variety is the spice of life, and it can be with your lifestyle goals too. Some aspects of routines are good to help you stick to your goals, but plan for some changes that are acceptable within your prediabetes care routine to keep things interesting too. Enrich your days by trying new things that are fun but still fit into your lifestyle plan. If you enjoy them, and they help your health, turn them into habits.

Tips to Make the Habit Stick

- Keep your eating plan tasty by trying out a new healthy restaurant or a new weekly recipe.
- Take a new exercise or dance class or walk a new route with your latest favorite music playing in your headphones to break up the monotony of your exercise plan.
- Make plans to do something different and fun for a date night or with your family or friends, or pick up that latest book you've been wanting to read.

91. *Don't* View Others' Good Intentions As Nagging, *Do* Communicate Clearly

When it comes to managing your prediabetes, do you feel as if your loved ones are always on your back? Pause and take a step back and realize they care about you and are concerned; however, their actions may be misguided. Use their positive support. They may sincerely want to help but just do not know how. Try to reframe nagging as a genuine concern from others and work out more concrete ways they can help you meet your goals.

Tips to Make the Habit Stick

- Talk to others respectfully, coolly, and calmly about specific ways they can help you. They should do things that you are comfortable with and that can help promote better blood sugars, weight, and health. Maybe help to you means going for a walk together or having them preprepping a healthy dinner while you are busy finishing a work deadline. Let them know the most effective ways to assist you.

- Take a moment to evaluate what your friends or family members are saying before reacting. Sometimes they may be pointing out things you don't see or are in denial about.

- Find ways to compromise and work together with the common goal of your health in mind. Consider their situation too. They may be stressed about your health situation and need some better self-care as well.

- If you need more assistance, seek out a therapist and/or a mediator in reaching common ground.

92. *Don't* Let Electronics Take over Your Life, *Do* Use Them Wisely

Technology is not going away—it is everywhere and anywhere, but in reasonable amounts it can be advantageous if you use it correctly. It can even help you work on your goals. Use technology sensibly and in small doses. Set limits for yourself on the amount of screen time you are engaging in to avoid getting caught up using technology (and sitting) for hours at a time.

Tips to Make the Habit Stick

- Using your smartphone is important for emergencies, to reach out to a friend when you are down, to play music when you are working out, or to get the latest application to track your steps and calories.

- Your computer, smartphone, or tablet is the gateway to the Internet to get educated about your condition, find new recipes, join an online support group, or keep your health journal in your efforts to manage your prediabetes.

- Beware of too much time with technology, though. It can lead to inactivity, interfere with your sleep, or take time away that could be spent enjoying fresh air outdoors as well as be replacing fun times or a great conversation with your family and friends. Find a balance.

93. *Don't* Try to Do Too Much at Once, *Do* Take a Few Steps at a Time

Once you have been diagnosed you may feel burdened with a long list of things you need to do and change. Rather than getting anxious and frazzled, make a list of what you want to achieve, prioritize what is important to do first, and break that down into smaller steps. Take things one step at a time to deal with the big picture of your health!

Tips to Make the Habit Stick

- Set small goals. Generally, you should work on no more than two or three specific goals at one time. This strategy prevents you from getting overwhelmed and allows you to master a goal before moving on to something else.
- Keep track of your goals and their outcomes to be aware of what you accomplished and what you still need to work on. This is where keeping a journal comes in handy.
- Often reaching out to a medical professional like a therapist or dietitian can help you with goal setting if you feel like you need some more assistance. They can help you set goals that will make you successful in controlling your prediabetes.

94. *Don't* Forget to Take Notes on Your Health, *Do* Keep a Journal or Diary

It can be very helpful to write about what you ate, how much you exercised, and/or what your goals and feelings are concerning your weight and blood sugar issues. Keeping a journal can be therapeutic, eye opening, and a great tool to use to help you and your medical team evaluate your prediabetes treatment plan.

Tips to Make the Habit Stick

- Make it as easy and convenient as possible to keep your journal. You may prefer a simple notebook, using a smartphone or tablet app, or buying a specially preformatted health journal.
- Try to keep the journal with you as much as possible so you can write down things as you go and so you won't forget details. The more complete it is, the more useful it becomes as a tool.
- Record your daily routine as it relates to food, exercise, and feelings.
- Look over your journal to evaluate progress and identify successes and areas for improvement.
- Bring your journal to your doctor appointments as a succinct and comprehensive way to keep the doctor apprised of your progress. Using it, she or he can decide if anything in your treatment plan needs to be adjusted.

95. *Don't* Disregard Sound Medical Advice, *Do* Listen to Your Medical Team

At times it can be tempting to take the easy way out and just be in denial about your prediabetes or look for overnight fixes. There are a lot of questionable diet plans, supplements, and treatment plans floating around on the Internet, television ads, and in health food stores. Realize that many of these have not been tested, are not scientifically proven to be effective, and they may even be unsafe. Studies have shown time and time again that lifestyle changes such as diet, exercise, weight loss, stress management, good sleep, and positive outlook and behaviors are the best way to manage prediabetes. If there was an amazing cure-all substitute, we would know about it by now. It may take time and effort to make lifestyle changes, but they will pay off and improve your overall health, not just your prediabetes.

Tips to Make the Habit Stick

- Listen to your doctor's recommendations and ask questions if you are unsure or don't feel comfortable with something.
- Bring any new supplements or treatment ideas to your medical team so you can evaluate them together to see if they are safe and feasible.
- Follow the tried-and-true lifestyle modifications for your prediabetes and consult your medical team before trying anything new or additional.

96. *Don't* Tune Out During Doctor's Appointments, *Do* Prepare for Them

Make the most of your time with your medical team since it is limited. Plan ahead to take advantage of your regular medical appointments and maximize your time with your medical team.

Tips to Make the Habit Stick

- Set a calendar reminder to keep track of appointments and arrive on time for them. Allow plenty of time to get there so you don't have to rush or arrive flustered.

- Take along your health diary and a list of questions or comments you may have for your practitioner.

- Bring menus or food labels, as well as a food diary, to your dietitian so she can provide clarification and suggestions.

- Having your partner, a family member, or a friend along at appointments can help you remember things. As well, they will remain in the know about your prediabetes treatment plan and get educated along with you.

- Don't forget to schedule regular follow-ups to stay up to date with reevaluating your condition and treatment goals.

97. *Don't* Beat Yourself Up, *Do* Learn from Your Successes and Failures

It is important to stay motivated and stick to your plan, but you have to realize you are not perfect. We all make mistakes; unexpected challenges come up, and sometimes we just get burned out and tired of dealing with a medical condition such as prediabetes. Realize that you will make mistakes, but look on the positive side that they are lessons to learn from.

Tips to Make the Habit Stick

- Give yourself permission to feel frustrated or disappointed, but not for too long so that you do not move on.
- Think about what led to your mistake and what you could have done differently or how you have been successful in the past and vow to try that the next time.
- Take a break with some deep breathing, an activity you enjoy, or try a walk or talk with a friend to take a mental break and then move on to better days.
- Journal your setbacks. Writing about the problem and ways you handled it versus how you could have solved it in a healthier way can be a good learning experience and a reference for you to reflect upon later.

98. *Don't* Set Overly Broad or Unrealistic Goals, *Do* Set Specific Goals

Be goal-oriented in the right way when it comes to your health and controlling your prediabetes. Remember to make your goals SMART: specific, measurable, action-oriented, realistic, and timely.

Tips to Make the Habit Stick

- Don't be too general. Goals like "I want better blood sugars" or "I want to lose weight," are too big and are not specific enough. They also have no time stamp on them. You need to break these goals down into smaller steps and plan how you are going to achieve them.
- Make your goals something you can live with. If you think, "I will never eat dessert ever again" or "I will exercise every day for one to two hours," these may seem too extreme and not be attainable or realistic.
- Be sure your goals are measurable, too, so that you can actually keep track of whether you met them or not, where your successes lie, and where there is room for improvement. For example: "I want to exercise for thirty minutes, three to five times a week" or "I want to eat two servings of vegetables per day" are more along the lines of smart goals.

99. *Don't* Get Away from Your Plan on Vacation, *Do* Enjoy Trips with Your Lifestyle Goals in Mind

Keeping up with your prediabetes treatment plan should be a lifelong goal, and you should work on it daily. With proper attention and planning you can still enjoy a change of pace while on a trip and still stay within the scope of what you are trying to achieve with your lifestyle changes. Keep your health agenda at the forefront while you travel to get the most out of your vacation and stick to your treatment goals.

Tips to Make the Habit Stick

- Create a basic schedule of your days so you can plan to work in activity and eat regular, healthy meals. Eat out sensibly, pack healthy snacks, and plan to move around on your trip as much as possible.
- Enjoy your downtime and opportunities to spend time with friends and family to reconnect and recharge. However, remind them of your goals and needs during the trip so they help you stay on track.

100. *Don't* Get Too Run Down, *Do* Take Time to Rest and Recharge

It's good to be busy and challenged, but doing too much can be overwhelming and lead to stress and burnout. Keep a healthy balance in your life, which includes making time for yourself, to help you keep on track with your lifestyle management and prediabetes treatment plan.

Tips to Make the Habit Stick

- Make sure to take breaks for regular meals/snacks, to drink fluids, and to move around.
- Get to bed early to get enough rest and give yourself time to breathe.
- If you need help with things at times with your crazy schedule, reach out to others and ask them for help in specific ways to lessen some of the burden.
- Don't overcommit yourself or take on more than is healthy for you to handle at work or in your personal life. That will invite stress.
- Make sure not to get so wrapped up in the hustle and bustle of the regular routine that you don't take time out to enjoy life, your hobbies, exercise, and time with family and friends.

Appendix A

A Grocery List for Good Health

Starches
- Whole-wheat or multigrain bread and English muffins
- Corn tortillas
- Low-carb tortilla
- High-fiber cereal (bran-based)
- Oatmeal
- Rice cakes
- Starchy vegetables and beans (corn, peas, pinto/garbanzo/black beans)
- Whole-wheat crackers

Fruits (fresh, **no** *canned or juices)*
- Bananas
- Melons
- Apples
- Berries
- Pears
- Oranges
- Grapes
- Avocados

Vegetables (fresh or fresh-frozen)
- Spinach/lettuce
- Mushrooms

- Tomatoes
- Zucchini
- Carrots
- Eggplants
- Celery
- Cauliflower
- Broccoli
- Asparagus
- Green beans
- Basil, Cilantro, Chives, Rosemary

Dairy

- Skim milk (light soymilk or unsweetened almond milk)
- Light yogurt
- Greek yogurt
- 2% cottage cheese
- 2% cheese slices and shredded cheese
- Light string cheese
- Light spreadable cheese wedges
- Fat-free or light cream cheese
- Fat-free half-and-half or soy/almond creamer (unsweetened)

Meat, Poultry, Meat Substitutes

- Chicken breasts
- Lean ground turkey
- Fish (halibut, salmon, tuna: fresh or frozen)
- Canned tuna (packed in water)
- Turkey breast
- Eggs or liquid egg whites

- Firm or extra-firm tofu
- Natural peanut butter or almond butter
- Hummus

Frozen Foods

- Frozen vegetables
- Frozen chicken breast and fish fillets (not breaded)
- Frozen edamame
- Protein "hamburger" style veggie burgers
- Low-sugar popsicles

Condiments, Canned Foods, Snack Foods, Beverages

- Light whipped butter or margarine
- Dijon mustard
- Vinegar (rice, balsamic, red wine)
- Salsa
- Tomato and marinara sauce
- Light mayonnaise
- Lower-sugar jam
- Low-sodium chicken or vegetable broth
- Nonstick cooking spray
- Olive oil
- Low-sodium soy sauce
- Spices (cinnamon, vanilla extract, pumpkin pie spice, garlic powder, onion powder, and other dried spices without salt)
- Nuts
- Light air-popped popcorn

Appendix B

Tips for Healthier Eating Out

Step One: Knowing the Right Approach

Planning ahead is essential for healthy dining out. Key points to remember are:

- Try to select a restaurant that you know has heart-healthy, low-fat menu options.
- When going to a new restaurant, try to preview the menu or call ahead to ask about the food choices and the possibility of accommodating your dietary needs.
- Have a low-fat, high-fiber snack (such as fruit and yogurt, raw veggies, or popcorn) to avoid feeling too hungry and prevent the temptation to overeat once you get there.
- Once you are there, read the menu carefully and beware of terms that signal high-fat and high-calorie items. Instead look for those that indicate foods with lower calories, low fat, and higher fiber.
- Don't be afraid to ask your server about menu specifics such as:

  - Methods of preparation (i.e., baked, steamed versus fried, battered).
  - Ingredients used (toppings, sauces, oil, cheeses).
  - Substitutions available (this ensures that you will know what to expect and won't have any surprises).

- To help control portions:

  - Order à la carte items, a few sides, or half portions for entrées.
  - Split large portions with friends or ask to take the second half home.
  - To round out the meal, start with a low-calorie beverage/low-fat appetizer and end with a healthy dessert.

- Keep a positive attitude and believe that you have the knowledge and the power to choose appropriate and healthful selections and control portions.

Step Two: Mastering the Menu: Terms to Be Familiar With

- Green-light words (these likely mean lower fat and/or lower calorie): steamed, baked, broiled, roasted, poached, garden fresh, grilled, lightly sautéed/stir-fried, boiled, skinless, plain/lean (menus may even highlight healthy/low-fat options).
- Red-light words (these often mean higher fat and/or higher calorie): buttered, fried, battered, creamed/creamy, breaded, au gratin, alfredo, cheesy, crispy/flaky, marinated, hollandaise, béarnaise, hash, pastry/fritter, parmigiana.
- Substitutions to suggest:

  - Insist on healthy methods of preparation. For example, ask for chicken skinless and baked instead of fried.
  - Be careful with toppings and sauces. Ask for fat-free or low-fat choices such as salsas, lemon juice, balsamic vinegar, red sauces,

teriyaki sauce, soy sauce (low sodium if available), mustard, ketchup, extra herbs/spices, jams or jellies, and raisins (some restaurants even offer lower-fat, low-calorie, and low-sodium versions of salad dressings, cheeses, and sour cream).

- If you must have a high-fat/calorie/sodium condiment, ask for it on the side to help control the amount you add. Try to use the following toppings sparingly: butter, cream sauces, full-fat salad dressings, sour cream, guacamole, cheeses, gravies, oils, whipped cream, salt, and soy sauce.

- Skip high-fat/calorie appetizers and sides and replace them with healthier ones:

  - Start with water, juices, fruit, salads, broth-based soups.
  - Ask for steamed vegetables, salads, pasta, brown rice, baked potatoes, whole-grain rolls instead of higher-fat sides such as French fries or onion rings.

- Pass on dessert if you are truly not hungry for it, but if you *need* to end with dessert then…

  - Try healthier, lower-calorie sweets such as fruit or berries with whipped cream.
  - Bring a low-fat treat with you (such as gum or hard candy).
  - Wait and eat a low-fat dessert at home, such as sugar-free Jell-O, low-fat frozen yogurt, or fruit.
  - If you must have the real thing…*share*, or at least halve the portion!

Step Three: Conquering Various Cuisines with the Right Choices

Italian
Starters/Sides:

- *Try:* minestrone soup, fresh vegetable salad, grilled vegetables (light olive oil), plain bread (or dip the bread in balsamic vinegar or small amounts of olive oil)
- *Skip:* fried calamari, cheese-based appetizers, bread with butter

Main Course:

- *Try:* pasta with red sauce or vegetables, grilled chicken/fish, small piece of pizza with light or no cheese and plenty of vegetable toppings), entrée-sized salads with grilled chicken or fish with balsamic vinegar, or dressing on the side
- *Skip*: veal/chicken/eggplant parmigiana, calzones, pizza with large amounts of cheese/meat, pasta with cream sauces/butter/cheese

Chinese/Japanese/Thai
Starters/Sides:

- *Try:* sashimi, green salad, miso soup or other broth-based soups with chicken/fish/tofu/vegetables, steamed chicken or vegetable dumplings, basil rolls, brown rice, steamed vegetables, low-sodium soy sauce or brown sauce on the side

- *Skip*: egg rolls, fried wontons, fried shrimp (tempura), beef or pork ribs, peanut or coconut sauces

Main Course:

- *Try*: steamed/broiled chicken, fish, tofu, or lean pork with vegetables and soy, brown or teriyaki sauce on the side, brown rice, soba noodles with veggies
- *Skip*: fried/battered beef, chicken, tofu, or seafood (tempura), fried rice, chow mein noodles in heavy oil, dishes with heavy coconut milk, duck, high-fat pork or red meat entrées

Mexican/Spanish

Starters/Sides:

- *Try*: gazpacho/black bean/tortilla soup, baked tortilla chips, whole-wheat flour or corn tortillas, vegetable salads, grilled vegetables (light oil), salsa, black or pinto beans (whole, no lard), turkey or vegetarian chili
- *Skip*: fried tortilla chips, guacamole, nachos, taquitos, salads with tostada/taco shells, refried beans with lard/cheese, fried plantains, menudo soup, meat chili

Main Course:

- *Try*: grilled chicken, fish, shrimp, or vegetable fajitas or soft tacos (hold the cheese/guacamole/sour cream), salsa/chili sauce, low-fat sour cream, entrée-sized salads with chicken, fish, black beans (dressing on the side)

- *Skip*: pork, beef or cheese enchiladas/burritos, fried/hard shell tacos, tostadas, taquitos, chimichangas, chorizo (pork sausage), added guacamole, cheese, sour cream

Indian
Starters/Sides:

- *Try*: broth-based soups (lentil, vegetable) leavened/baked breads (whole wheat if available) like naan/kulcha/chapati, spiced vegetables/salads, lentils/potatoes cooked in tomato or broth, low-fat yogurt, chutney, dahl (lentil) sauce
- *Skip*: coconut soup, fried breads (paratha, poori) coconut/nut-based sauces, fried rice/potato/vegetable dishes, fried or cheese-based appetizers

Main Course:

- *Try*: tandoori/masala roasted/baked chicken or seafood, lentil/chickpea dishes with vegetables in spiced broth or tomatoes
- *Skip*: all dishes that are fried or have cream curry/cheese-based sauces

Mediterranean
Starters/Sides/Main Course:

- *Try*: vegetable salads, grilled vegetables (light/no oil), small amounts of hummus, baba ganoush, whole-wheat pita bread, tabbouleh, dolmas (grape leaves) stuffed with vegetables/rice,

broth-based lentil or vegetable soups, kalamata olives, chicken/
seafood/vegetable kabobs/gyros
- *Skip*: dolmas with feta cheese/lamb, fried falafel, pastries with
  cheese/meat, moussaka (eggplant with cheese) beef/lamb
  kabob/gyros

American/Diners
Starters/Sides:

- *Try*: vegetable salads, steamed vegetables, broth-based soups
  (vegetable, chicken, bean), low-fat cottage cheese, fruit salad,
  baked potato, whole-grain bread or rolls, shrimp cocktail, vegetarian chili
- *Skip*: cream- and cheese-based soups, fried appetizers (chicken
  wings/fingers, onion rings, French fries), creamed or buttered
  vegetables, coleslaw, potato salad

Main Course:

- *Try*: entrée-sized salads with added beans, plain tuna, egg
  whites, grilled chicken or fish (light dressing, balsamic/red
  wine vinegar or dressing on side), grilled vegetables, turkey
  or chicken sandwiches on whole-grain bread, turkey or veggie
  burgers on whole-wheat bun, grilled or baked chicken/turkey/
  seafood with veggies and brown rice
- *Skip*: chef or Caesar salad, beef/pastrami sandwiches, chicken/
  tuna/egg salad with mayo

Breakfast Dishes
Starters/Sides/Main Course:

- *Try*: fresh fruit, non- or low-fat cottage cheese or yogurt, whole-grain toast, wheat English muffin or half bagel with jam or light cream cheese, sliced tomatoes, turkey or Canadian bacon/turkey sausage, egg-white omelets with veggies, bran or oat cold cereal with skim milk, oatmeal with skim milk and chopped nuts
- *Skip:* whole-milk yogurt/cottage cheese, regular muffins, pastries, doughnuts, white bagels/English muffins with butter/ regular cream cheese, hash browns/fried potatoes, granola, beef/pork sausage, biscuits, gravy, waffles, pancakes, whole-egg dishes

Appendix C

Online Prediabetes/Diabetes Education Resources

General Information

dLife

An interactive diabetes website that includes diabetes information, tips for healthy eating, a recipe bank, and a diabetic community.

www.dlife.com

National Institute of Diabetes and Digestive and Kidney Disease

A site for general diabetes information where brochures and articles can be downloaded.

www.niddk.nih.gov

Taking Control of Your Diabetes

Established by endocrinologist Dr. Steven Edelman, this unique series of national conferences offers people with diabetes a day of education and connection with others. You can find a conference near you on their website or learn from some of their many videos and features online.

www.tcoyd.org

Joslin Diabetes Center

The world-renowned Boston-based Joslin Diabetes Center is a leading diabetes care and research facility. They also have accredited satellite programs throughout the US and fantastic online resources.

www.joslin.org

National Diabetes Education Program (NDEP)

The NDEP helps translate the latest diabetes research into practical information for people with diabetes. Their website features many free, downloadable publications.
www.ndep.nih.gov

US National Library of Medicine and National Institutes of Health

This site has research, references, interactive tutorials, consumer materials, and guidebooks to download or order online.
https://medlineplus.gov/diabetes.html

Diet and Nutrition

American Diabetes Association

This site, maintained by the recognized authority on diabetes, is dedicated to providing up-to-date diabetes information, researching findings, and advocating for people with diabetes.
www.diabetes.org

Ask the Dietitian

Joanne Larsen, MS, RD, LD, maintains this site. You can use it to post specific diet-related questions or read the answers to questions from other visitors.
www.dietitian.com

Cornerstones4Care

An interactive website with menu-planning tools, articles, and a free diabetes ebook that you can download.
www.cornerstones4care.com

University of Sydney's Glycemic Index

This internationally recognized center of nutritional research offers a full searchable database of glycemic index and glycemic load values.
www.glycemicindex.com

USDA ChooseMyPlate

A site developed by the US Department of Agriculture that discusses the MyPlate tool, which reviews and illustrates the five food groups and is the USDA's latest food guide symbol. It reviews all the food groups in detail, discusses portions and healthy choices, and there is also a section on physical activity. Recipes and other tools are available on the site as well.
www.choosemyplate.gov

Cornerstones4Care Carb Counting and Meal Planning

A comprehensive tool developed by Novo Nordisk to help patients with carbohydrate counting and meal planning.
www.novomedlink.com/content/dam/novonordisk/novomedlink/resources/generaldocuments/CountingCarbandMeal_EG.pdf

MyFitnessPal

A site (also available as an app) that enables you to track food and physical activity and also includes an online community element for social support.
www.myfitnesspal.com

SparkPeople

Free online site available for calorie and exercise tracking with a strong online support network as well as educational articles and videos.
www.sparkpeople.com

Fitness and Exercise

Dance Out Diabetes

A San Francisco–based organization with a mission to "prevent and manage diabetes through dance, education, support and increased access to care."
www.danceoutdiabetes.org

American Council of Exercise (ACE)

A nonprofit organization that certifies fitness professionals and promotes safe and effective physical activity. The ACE Healthy Living Blog area of their website offers great tips for exercising and healthy eating.
www.acefitness.org/education-and-resources/lifestyle/blog/

Kids and Teens with Diabetes

Diabetes Education and Camping Association (DECA)
Camp is a great way for children to learn more about caring for their condition, to meet others like them, and to have fun doing it. Many camps now offer type 2 programs for kids. Search DECA's extensive database for a camp near you.
www.diabetescamps.org

Alliance for a Healthier Generation
Helpful website offering practical ideas to parents and children working toward healthy lifestyle behaviors.
www.healthiergeneration.org

Advocacy Organizations

American Diabetes Association (ADA)
The ADA sets clinical diabetes standards for US physicians and also acts on behalf of diabetes patients to fund research and fight discrimination. Visit their website or call 1-800-DIABETES for more information.
www.diabetes.org

Diabetes Canada
Formerly the Canadian Diabetes Association, this organization is "leading the fight against diabetes by helping people with diabetes live healthy lives while working to find the cure."
www.diabetes.ca

Support Groups and Communities

Dear Janis, with CDE/RD Janis Roszler
Certified diabetes educator, marriage and family therapist, and registered dietitian Janis Roszler oversees this excellent site that features a small but active diabetes forum.
www.dearjanis.com

Diabetes Daily

A community-focused site featuring blogs, groups, chats, and online workshops. Run by Elizabeth Zabell and David Edelman.
www.diabetesdaily.com

DiabetesSisters

Diabetes activist Brandy Barnes launched this diabetes community in 2008 as a safe place for women to talk about the unique diabetes issues they face. In addition to the online community forums, you can find a local or national meeting, sign up for the mentoring "Sister Match" program, or read some of the featured blogs and expert commentary.
www.diabetessisters.org

Divabetic

Geared toward women but open to all, this grassroots organization was founded by Max Szadek. Max was an assistant to singer Luther Vandross, who passed away from type 2 diabetes–related complications in 2005. Divabetic strives to make the process of learning about diabetes self-management fun and enjoyable.
https://divabetic.org

TuDiabetes

Run by the Diabetes Hands Foundation, this vibrant community site offers lively discussion, blogs, groups, videos, and special promotions.
https://tudiabetes.org

Appendix D

Bibliography

Chapter 1

Rhoades, R., and Pflanzer, R. (1992). *Human Physiology.* Fort Worth, TX: Saunders College Publishing.

Promeet, D. (2009, May 4). Islets of Langerhans. Retrieved from www.britannica.com/science/islets-of-Langerhans/.

Blood Glucose Control Studies for Type 1 Diabetes: DCCT and EDIC. Retrieved from www.niddk.nih.gov/about-niddk/research-areas/diabetes/blood-glucose-control-studies-type-1-diabetes-dcct-edic.

Hyperosmolar Hyperglycemic Nonketotic Syndrome (HHNS). (2013, August 21). Retrieved from www.diabetes.org/living-with-diabetes/complications/hyperosmolar-hyperglycemic.html.

Assessing Your Weight and Health Risk. Retrieved from www.nhlbi.nih.gov/health/educational/lose_wt/risk.htm.

DKA (Ketoacidosis) & Ketones. (2013, August 21). Retrieved from www.diabetes.org/living-with-diabetes/complications/ketoacidosis-dka.html.

Gebel, E. (2012, February). Prediabetes and You. *Diabetes Forecast.* Retrieved from www.diabetesforecast.org/2012/feb/prediabetes-and-you.html#.

Chapter 2

Statistics About Diabetes. (2018, March 22). Retrieved from www.diabetes.org/diabetes-basics/statistics/.

Diabetes Statistics. (2017, September). Retrieved from www.niddk.nih.gov/health-information/health-statistics/diabetes-statistics.

Standards of Medical Care in Diabetes—2018. Abridged for Primary Care Providers. American Diabetes Association. *Diabetes Care* 41(Suppl.1): S1-S159. Retrieved from http://clinical.diabetesjournals.org/content/diaclin/early/2017/12/07/cd17-0119.full.pdf.

Cardiovascular Disease and Diabetes. (2015, August 30). Retrieved from www.heart.org/en/health-topics/diabetes/why-diabetes-matters/cardiovascular-disease--diabetes.

Zhilei, S. et al. (2015). Sleep Duration and Risk of Type 2 Diabetes: A Meta-analysis of Prospective Studies. *Diabetes Care* 38(3), 529–537. Retrieved from http://care.diabetesjournals.org/content/38/3/529.

Dinsmoor, R. (2017, September 11). Metformin. Retrieved from www.diabetesselfmanagement.com/diabetes-resources/definitions/metformin/.

The Diabetes Prevention Program. (2002, December). *Diabetes Care* 25(12): 2,165–2,171. Retrieved from http://care.diabetesjournals.org/content/25/12/2165.

Chapter 3

Blanco, C. (2014, May 8). The principal sources of William James' idea of habit. *Frontiers in Human Neuroscience* (274). Retrieved from www.ncbi.nlm.nih.gov/pmc/articles/PMC4077119/.

Duhigg, C. (2012). *The Power of Habit: Why We Do What We Do in Life and Business.* New York: Random House Trade Paperbacks.

James, W. (1914). *Habit* [electronic version]. Retrieved from https://archive.org/details/habitjam00jameuoft.

Neal, D. et al. (2006). Habits—A Repeat Performance. *Current Directions in Psychological Science* 15(4), 198–202. Retrieved from https://dornsife.usc.edu/assets/sites/208/docs/Neal.Wood.Quinn.2006.pdf.

Jager, W. (2003). Breaking 'bad habits': a dynamical perspective on habit formation and change [electronic version]. Retrieved from www.rug.nl/staff/w.jager/jager_habits_chapter_2003.pdf.

Gardner, B. (2015). A review and analysis of the use of 'habit' in understanding, predicting and influencing health-related behaviour. *Health Psychology Review* 9(3), 277–295. Retrieved from www.ncbi.nlm.nih.gov/pmc/articles/PMC4566897/.

Verhoeven, A. et al. (2014). Identifying the 'if' for 'if-then' plans: combining implementation intentions with cue-monitoring targeting unhealthy snacking behaviour. *Psychology & Health* 29(12), 1,476–1,492. Retrieved from www.ncbi.nlm.nih.gov/pubmed/25099386.

Lanciego, J. et al. (2012). Functional Neuroanatomy of the Basal Ganglia. *Cold Spring Harbor Perspectives in Medicine* 2(12). Retrieved from www.ncbi.nlm.nih.gov/pmc/articles/PMC3543080/#!po=43.3884.

Seger, C. et al. (2011). A Critical Review of Habit Learning and the Basal Ganglia. *Frontiers in Systems Neuroscience* 5(66). Retrieved from www.ncbi.nlm.nih.gov/pmc/articles/PMC3163829/.

Wood, W. et al. (2016). Psychology of Habit. *Annual Review of Psychology* (67), 289-314. Retrieved from www.annualreviews.org/doi/10.1146/annurev-psych-122414-033417.

Gardner, B. et al. (2012). Making health habitual: the psychology of 'habit-formation' and general practice. *British Journal of General Practice* 62(605), 664–666. Retrieved from www.ncbi.nlm.nih.gov/pmc/articles/PMC3505409/.

Schwabe, L. et al. (2009). Stress Prompts Habit Behavior in Humans. *Journal of Neuroscience* 29(22), 7,191–7,198. Retrieved from www.jneurosci.org/content/29/22/7191.full.

Cleo, G. et al. (2018). Participant experiences of two successful habit-based weight-loss interventions in Australia: a qualitative study. *British Medical Journal Open* 8(5). Retrieved from www.ncbi.nlm.nih.gov/pmc/articles/PMC5988089/.

Graybiel, A. (1998). The Basal Ganglia and Chunking of Action Repertoires. *Neurobiology of Learning and Memory* 70(1-2), 119–136. Retrieved from www-edlab.cs.umass.edu/cs691jj/NBLM_Graybiel.pdf.

Cleo, G. et al. (2018). Habit-based interventions for weight loss maintenance in adults with overweight and obesity: a randomized controlled trial. *International Journal of Obesity*, April 23. Retrieved from www.ncbi.nlm.nih.gov/pubmed/29686382.

Changing Your Habits for Better Health. (2017, May). Retrieved from www.niddk.nih.gov/health-information/diet-nutrition/changing-habits-better-health.

Butterworth, S. et al. (2006). Effect of motivational interviewing-based health coaching on employees' physical and mental status. *Journal of Occupational Health Psychology* 11(4), 358–365. Retrieved from www.researchgate.net/profile/Michael_Leo/publication/6737390_Effect_of_motivational_interviewing-based_health_coaching_on_employees'_physical_and_mental_status/links/0fcfd50a27e2d2f505000000.pdf.

Pirzadeh, A. et al. (2015). Applying Transtheoretical Model to Promote Physical Activities Among Women. *Iranian Journal of Psychiatry and Behavioral Sciences* 9(4), e1580. Retrieved from www.ncbi.nlm.nih.gov/pmc/articles/PMC4733300/.

Chapter 4

Standards of Medical Care in Diabetes—2018. Abridged for Primary Care Providers. American Diabetes Association. *Diabetes Care* 41(Suppl.1): S1–S159. Retrieved from http://clinical.diabetesjournals.org/content/diaclin/early/2017/12/07/cd17-0119.full.pdf.

Fats. (2015, August 13). Retrieved from www.diabetes.org/food-and-fitness/food/what-can-i-eat/making-healthy-food-choices/fats-and-diabetes.html.

Changes to the Nutrition Facts Label. (2018, June 28). Retrieved from www.fda.gov/Food/GuidanceRegulation/GuidanceDocumentsRegulatoryInformation/LabelingNutrition/ucm385663.htm.

Chapter 5

Batchelor, M. (2016). Health consequences of inactivity and approaches to overcome sedentary behaviors. *On the Cutting Edge* 36(6), 4–7.

Standards of Medical Care in Diabetes—2018. Abridged for Primary Care Providers. American Diabetes Association. *Diabetes Care* 41(Suppl.1): S1–S159. Retrieved from http://clinical.diabetesjournals.org/content/diaclin/early/2017/12/07/cd17-0119.full.pdf.

Colberg, S. (2016). Supporting early adoption of exercise in adults with type 2 diabetes: what the nutrition professional needs to know. *On the Cutting Edge* (36)6, 15–21.

Isaak, S. et al. (2016). Fitness tools and technology: making a difference for our patients with diabetes. *On the Cutting Edge* 36(6), 34–36.

Hayes, C. (2001). *The I Hate to Exercise Book for People with Diabetes*. Alexandria, VA: Self-pub, American Diabetes Association.

Forberg, C. (2015). *A Small Guide to Losing Big*. Napa, CA: Flavor First LLC.

Padayachee, C. et al. (2015, July 25). Exercise guidelines for gestational diabetes mellitus. *World Journal of Diabetes* 6(8), 1,033–1,044. Retrieved from www.ncbi.nlm.nih.gov/pmc/articles/PMC4515443/.

Chapter 6

Adult Obesity Facts. (2018, August 13). Retrieved from www.cdc.gov/obesity/data/adult.html.

Standards of Medical Care in Diabetes—2018. Abridged for Primary Care Providers. American Diabetes Association. (2018). *Diabetes Care* 41(Suppl.1): S1–S159. Retrieved from http://clinical.diabetesjournals.org/content/diaclin/early/2017/12/07/cd17-0119.full.pdf.

Pietrzykowska, N. (2018). Benefits of 5–10 Percent Weight-Loss. Retrieved from www.obesityaction.org/educational-resources/resource-articles-2/general-articles/benefits-of-5-10-percent-weight-loss.

Adachi, Y. (2005). Behavior Therapy for Obesity. JMAJ 48(11), 539–544. Retrieved from www.med.or.jp/english/pdf/2005_11/539_544.pdf.

Forberg, C. (2015). *A Small Guide to Losing Big*. Napa, CA: Flavor First LLC.

van Strien, T. (2018, April 25). Causes of Emotional Eating and Matched Treatment of Obesity. *Current Diabetes Reports* 18(6), 35. Retrieved from www.ncbi.nlm.nih.gov/pmc/articles/PMC5918520/.

Weight loss: Gain control of emotional eating. (2015, October 3). Retrieved from www.mayoclinic.org/healthy-lifestyle/weight-loss/in-depth/weight-loss/art-20047342.

Parretti, H. et al. (2015, September). Efficacy of water preloading before main meals as a strategy for weight loss in primary care patients with obesity: RCT. *Obesity* 23(9), 1,785–1,791. Retrieved from https://onlinelibrary.wiley.com/doi/abs/10.1002/oby.21167.

Jakubowicz, D. et al. (2013). High caloric intake at breakfast vs. dinner differentially influences weight loss of overweight and obese women. *Obesity* 21(12) 2504–2512. Retrieved from www.ncbi.nlm.nih.gov/pubmed/23512957.

Panchal, SK et al. (2018). Capsaicin in Metabolic Syndrome. *Nutrients* 10(5), E630. Retrieved from www.ncbi.nlm.nih.gov/pubmed/29772784.

Chapter 7

Stress. (2018). Retrieved from www.mentalhealthamerica.net/conditions/stress.

Stress. (2013, June 7). Retrieved from www.diabetes.org/living-with-diabetes/complications/mental-health/stress.html.

Listening to the warning signs of stress. (2018). Retrieved from www.apa.org/helpcenter/stress-signs.aspx.

Chen, S. et al. (2016). Association of depression with pre-diabetes, undiagnosed diabetes, and previously diagnosed diabetes: a meta-analysis. *Endocrine* 53(1), 35–46. Retrieved from www.ncbi.nlm.nih.gov/pubmed/26832340.

Ghorbani, A. et al. (2015). Association of Sleep Quality and Waking Time with Prediabetes: The Qazvin Metabolic Diseases Study, Iran. *Sleep Disorders* (480742). Retrieved from www.ncbi.nlm.nih.gov/pubmed/26351585.

Hung, H. et al. (2013). The Association between Self-Reported Sleep Quality and Metabolic Syndrome. *PLOS One*. Retrieved from http://journals.plos.org/plosone/article?id=10.1371/journal.pone.0054304.

Sleep Deprivation and Deficiency—Why Is Sleep Important? Retrieved from www.nhlbi.nih.gov/node/4605.

Hirshkowitz, M. et al. (2015). National Sleep Foundation's sleep time duration recommendations: methodology and results summary. *Sleep Health* 1(1), 40–43. Retrieved from www.sleephealthjournal.org/article/S2352-7218%2815%2900015-7/fulltext.

What is Good Quality Sleep? (2017, January 23). Retrieved from https://sleepfoundation.org/press-release/what-good-quality-sleep.

1 in 3 adults don't get enough sleep. (2016, February 18). Retrieved from www.cdc.gov/media/releases/2016/p0215-enough-sleep.html.

Roth, T. (2007). Insomnia: Definition, Prevalence, Etiology, and Consequences. *Journal of Clinical Sleep Medicine* 3(5 Suppl), S7–S10. Retrieved from www.ncbi.nlm.nih.gov/pmc/articles/PMC1978319/.

Lee, A. et al. (2018). Diabetes Distress and Glycemic Control: The Buffering Effect of Autonomy Support From Important Family Members and Friends. *Diabetes Care* 41(6), 1,157–1,163. Retrieved from http://care.diabetesjournals.org/content/41/6/1157.

Wang, X. et al. (2014). Social support moderates stress effects on depression. *International Journal of Mental Health Systems* 8(41). Retrieved from https://ijmhs.biomedcentral.com/articles/10.1186/1752-4458-8-41.

Rad, G.S. et al. (2013). Importance of social support in diabetes care. *Journal of Education and Health Promotion* 2(62). Retrieved from www.ncbi.nlm.nih.gov/pmc/articles/PMC3908488/.

Akour, A. et al. (2018). Association of Oxytocin with Glucose Intolerance and Inflammation Biomarkers in Metabolic Syndrome Patients with and without Prediabetes. *Review of Diabetic Studies*. Winter 14(4), 364–371. Retrieved from www.ncbi.nlm.nih.gov/pubmed/29590229.

Schumann, K. et al. (2011). Evidence-Based Behavioral Treatments for Diabetes: Problem-Solving Therapy. *Diabetes Spectrum* 24(2), 64–69. Retrieved from http://spectrum.diabetesjournals.org/content/24/2/64.

AADE7 Self-Care Behaviors™. (2018). Retrieved from www.diabeteseducator.org/living-with-diabetes/aade7-self-care-behaviors.

Problem Solving. (2018). Retrieved from www.diabeteseducator.org/living-with-diabetes/aade7-self-care-behaviors/problem-solving.

What is a CDE? (2018). Retrieved from www.ncbde.org/certification_info/what-is-a-cde/.

Zhu, L. et al. (2012). Circadian Rhythm Sleep Disorders. *Neurologic Clinics* 30(4), 1,167–1,191. Retrieved from www.ncbi.nlm.nih.gov/pmc/articles/PMC3523094/.

Horne J. et al. (1983). Exercise and sleep: body-heating effects. *Sleep* 6(1), 36–46. Retrieved from https://www.ncbi.nlm.nih.gov/pubmed/6844796.

Passos, G. et al. (2011). Effects of moderate aerobic exercise training on chronic primary insomnia. *Sleep Medicine* 12(10), 1,018–1,027. Retrieved from www.ncbi.nlm.nih.gov/pubmed/22019457.

Healthy Sleep Tips (2018). Retrieved from https://sleepfoundation.org/sleep-tools-tips/healthy-sleep-tips.

Shekhar, S. et al. (2018). Effect of 6 Months of Meditation on Blood Sugar, Glycosylated Hemoglobin, and Insulin Levels in Patients of Coronary Artery Disease. *International Journal of Yoga* 11(2), 122–128. Retrieved from www.ncbi.nlm.nih.gov/pmc/articles/PMC5934947/.

Noureldein, M. et al. (2018, January). Homeostatic effect of laughter on diabetic cardiovascular complications: The myth turned to fact. *Diabetes Research and Clinical Practice* (135), 111–119. Retrieved from www.ncbi.nlm.nih.gov/pubmed/29162513.

Yeung, J. et al. (2017). Volunteering and health benefits in general adults: cumulative effects and forms. *BMC Public Health* 18(8). Retrieved from https://bmcpublichealth.biomedcentral.com/articles/10.1186/s12889-017-4561-8.

Appendix E

US/Metric Conversion Chart

VOLUME CONVERSIONS

US Volume Measure	Metric Equivalent
⅛ teaspoon	0.5 milliliter
¼ teaspoon	1 milliliter
½ teaspoon	2 milliliters
1 teaspoon	5 milliliters
½ tablespoon	7 milliliters
1 tablespoon (3 teaspoons)	15 milliliters
2 tablespoons (1 fluid ounce)	30 milliliters
¼ cup (4 tablespoons)	60 milliliters
⅓ cup	80 milliliters
½ cup (4 fluid ounces)	125 milliliters
⅔ cup	160 milliliters
¾ cup (6 fluid ounces)	180 milliliters
1 cup (16 tablespoons)	250 milliliters
1 pint (2 cups)	500 milliliters
1 quart (4 cups)	1 liter (about)

WEIGHT CONVERSIONS

US Weight Measure	Metric Equivalent
½ ounce	15 grams
1 ounce	30 grams
2 ounces	60 grams
3 ounces	85 grams
¼ pound (4 ounces)	115 grams
½ pound (8 ounces)	225 grams
¾ pound (12 ounces)	340 grams
1 pound (16 ounces)	454 grams

OVEN TEMPERATURE CONVERSIONS

Degrees Fahrenheit	Degrees Celsius
200 degrees F	95 degrees C
250 degrees F	120 degrees C
275 degrees F	135 degrees C
300 degrees F	150 degrees C
325 degrees F	160 degrees C
350 degrees F	180 degrees C
375 degrees F	190 degrees C
400 degrees F	205 degrees C
425 degrees F	220 degrees C
450 degrees F	230 degrees C

BAKING PAN SIZES

American	Metric
8 × 1½ inch round baking pan	20 × 4 cm cake tin
9 × 1½ inch round baking pan	23 × 3.5 cm cake tin
11 × 7 × 1½ inch baking pan	28 × 18 × 4 cm baking tin
13 × 9 × 2 inch baking pan	30 × 20 × 5 cm baking tin
2 quart rectangular baking dish	30 × 20 × 3 cm baking tin
15 × 10 × 2 inch baking pan	38 × 25 × 5 cm baking tin (Swiss roll tin)
9 inch pie plate	22 × 4 or 23 × 4 cm pie plate
7 or 8 inch springform pan	18 or 20 cm springform or loose bottom cake tin
9 × 5 × 3 inch loaf pan	23 × 13 × 7 cm or 2 lb narrow loaf or pâté tin
1½ quart casserole	1.5 liter casserole
2 quart casserole	2 liter casserole

Index

ABOUT THE AUTHOR

Marie Feldman has been a registered dietitian for more than nineteen years and has worked as a certified diabetes educator for ten of them. She received her bachelor's degree in clinical dietetics at UC Berkeley and has been an outpatient dietitian at other institutions including Memorial Sloan Kettering and Cedars-Sinai. She enjoys providing medical nutrition therapy and education to adults, namely in the areas of weight management and diabetes. In addition, she has served as a research department manager and helped facilitate more than thirty industry-based clinical trials, primarily with a focus on diabetes and cardiovascular disease. She has maintained her nutrition blog, NourishYouDelicious.Blogspot.com, for almost ten years and recently published a diabetes cookbook, *The Big Book of Diabetic Recipes*.